RAPTURE

ART'S SEDUCTION BY FASHION SINCE 1970
CHRIS TOWNSEND

WITH 172 ILLUSTRATIONS, 165 IN COLOUR

Thames & Hudson

DESIGN ALEXANDER BOXILL

FIRST PUBLISHED IN THE UNITED KINGDOM
IN 2002 BY THAMES & HUDSON LTD
181A HIGH HOLBORN
LONDON WC1V 7QX

WWW.THAMESANDHUDSON.COM

© CHRIS TOWNSEND 2002

THIS PUBLICATION ACCOMPANIES AN EXHIBITION
RAPTURE
ART'S SEDUCTION BY FASHION SINCE 1970

10 OCTOBER – 23 DECEMBER 2002

BARBICAN GALLERY
BARBICAN CENTRE
SILK STREET
LONDON EC2Y 8DS
WWW.BARBICAN.ORG.UK

BARBICAN ART GALLERIES ARE OWNED, FUNDED
AND MANAGED BY THE CORPORATION OF LONDON

EXHIBITION CURATED CHRIS TOWNSEND
EXHIBITION ORGANISED JANE ALISON, CURATOR;
CATHERINE WOOD, EXHIBITION ORGANISER;
KATHERINE OLIVER, CURATORIAL ASSISTANT
(BARBICAN ART GALLERIES)

barbican

FOR OVER HALF A CENTURY, LAVAZZA HAS
STRONGLY BELIEVED IN THE VALUE OF THE
BOND FORGED BETWEEN COMMUNICATIONS
AND ART, AND HAS ENHANCED ARTISTS'
FREEDOM TO CREATE WORKS OF ART IN THE
FIELDS OF PHOTOGRAPHY, DESIGN, CINEMA,
NEW TECHNOLOGIES AND FASHION.

TODAY LAVAZZA IS THE PROUD PARTNER IN
THE EXHIBITION 'RAPTURE' AND SHARES ITS
DEDICATION TO FREE EXPRESSION THROUGH
ART BY LEADING CONTEMPORARY ARTISTS.

LAVAZZA
ITALY'S FAVOURITE COFFEE

LUIGI LAVAZZA
CORSO NOVARA 59
10154 TORINO, ITALY
WWW.LAVAZZA.COM

BRITISH LIBRARY CATALOGUING-IN-PUBLICATION DATA
A CATALOGUE RECORD FOR THIS BOOK IS AVAILABLE
FROM THE BRITISH LIBRARY

ISBN 0-500-28383-4

PRINTED AND BOUND IN ITALY BY CONTI TIPOCOLOR

Frank Moore
To Die For, 1997
Oil on canvas on featherboard
with mirror frame

The iconic face of fashion in our
time – Kate Moss – transformed
simultaneously into mythological
character and fashion's most
distinctive logo; an image that
encapsulates the compressions
and convergences between
fashion and contemporary art.

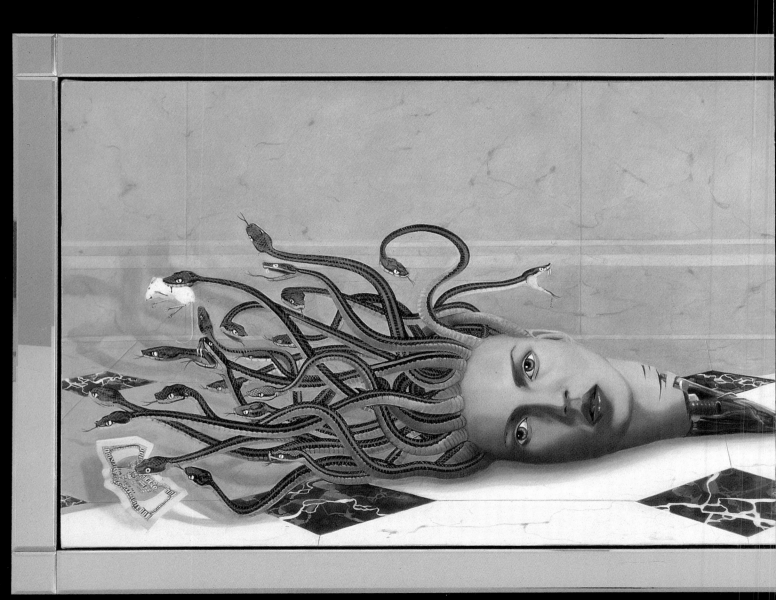

INTRODUCTION

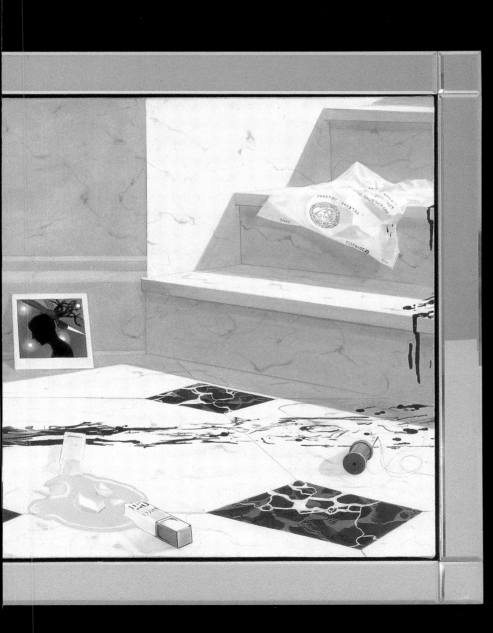

I am standing in the back room of a gallery in New York's SoHo, contemplating a painting by the American artist Frank Moore. Entitled *To Die For*, this work rephrases in contemporary terms the classical myth of the Medusa, the snake-haired Gorgon who turned all who confronted her to stone. Moore has depicted the severed head lying on a bloodstained marble floor, its serpentine tresses still writhing, blankly returning the viewer's gaze yet able still to petrify, to freeze the spectator for perpetuity. As if to explain, in case we have forgotten the narrative that brought us – artist, spectator, mythological monster – to this moment, Moore incorporates a self-referential compression of time, a photograph of the moment at which the decapitating knife bore down upon Medusa's neck.

This Gorgon, however, is no anonymous victim of an unseen slayer. Moore has painted his subject with the face of the English fashion model Kate Moss – an iconic visage of our time, a face that, simultaneously mundane and staggeringly beautiful, does indeed possess the power to arrest our vision, to stop us in our tracks; a face that, in a very Freudian way, can petrify us. But Moore's choice of Moss is not as simple as that. This painting – this resort to an antique medium in the modern moment – is not merely concerned with the arresting power of the gaze, no matter on whom it is turned. Rather, *To Die For*, and for that matter my engagement with it in this particular quarter of New York, encapsulates and compresses the complex relationships of fashion and art, both in our time as an apparently novel phenomenon, and in history as a phenomenon we endlessly repeat.

Read as a history painting – a historical subject inserted into classical fantasy – this painting comes with its own history. *To Die For* was commissioned by the fashion designer Gianni Versace in 1997, shortly before his murder. The painting is bound to fashion by its model subject, and also by the desire that brought it into existence. Its iconicity thus becomes a kind of double-bind: that Moore should paint Moss as Medusa, for Versace, is to answer fashion's need to see itself reflected in the mirror of art – as the Gorgon saw herself, momentarily, fatally, in Perseus' burnished shield. The star model is placed in the foreground as the arresting symbol of to-die-for clothes: Moss becomes Versace's trade-mark, though the author never lived to see it written. *To Die For* suggests that in fashion who's dying, and for what, is a rather more complex set of transactions than the exchange of credit for this season's signature dress.

The Versace logo is still Medusa's head, its stylized glare repeated on the buttons and myriad garments and accessories in fashion stores, new, and in wardrobes, maybe used or else still invested with the promise of use. These garments and accessories are made new each season, but the Versace signature upon them remains a constant; a reminder not only of fashion's capability to transfix us, to render us its victims, but – as I reflected on first looking at a painting completed too late to

**Gianni Versace
Gold Medusa watch,
1991**

The image of horror – the
Medusa's petrifying visage – is
transmuted into an ostentatious
symbol of luxury and a very
particular form of taste.
The classical motif undergoes
a process of condensation
and transference; a prophecy
perhaps of the future of art's
own signs within fashion.

Looking at *To Die For* in SoHo enfolds
Moore's painting and this critique, its
outline scribbled into a tiny black
notebook gifted by a newly launched
fashion magazine, into a register of art
and fashion's shared histories and myths,
in which 'Absolut Versace' and 'Absolut Ofili'
are images of defining moments. South
of Houston – SoHo, downtown Manhattan
bounded by Varick, Canal Street, Lafayette
and East Houston – is now a geographic
space that, in its social realities, manifests
the same interweaving as Frank Moore
mythifies in the space of his painting.
The season-to-season turnover of styles
and designs – fashion's reinvention of its
own and other people's pasts – is taking
place in the streets immediately outside
this gallery. In Helmut Lang, Comme des
Garçons, Agnès b, contemplations figured
as much upon haptic sensuality as the
fractal scrutinies of visual seduction are
accompanied by ambient minimalism,
muted baroque or barcode techno, even
as I engage in the quiet and distanced
consideration that is the proper relationship
of art and its critics. In the mid-1990s SoHo
became the one place to open a store if you
were a fashion magnate with your eye on
the balance sheet and pretensions to a
status commensurate with the architecture
and furnishings of both your head office and
your ego. It became a territory to die for.

This gallery, on the upper floor of what
passes in New York for a historic building,
now feels out of place – like spring's so-
last-season shirt worn within the white-
heat of this winter's must-have coat.
Twenty-five years ago, when this gallery

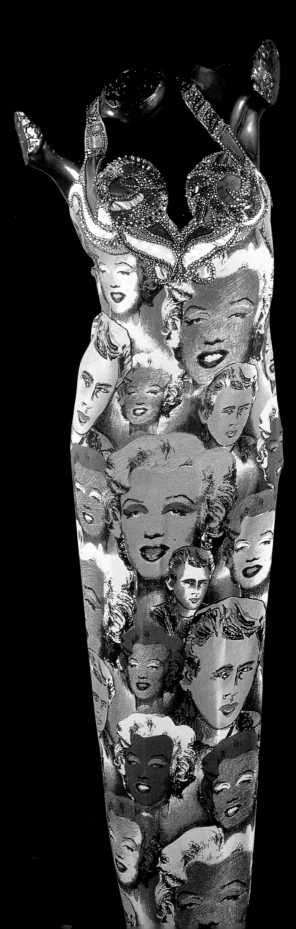

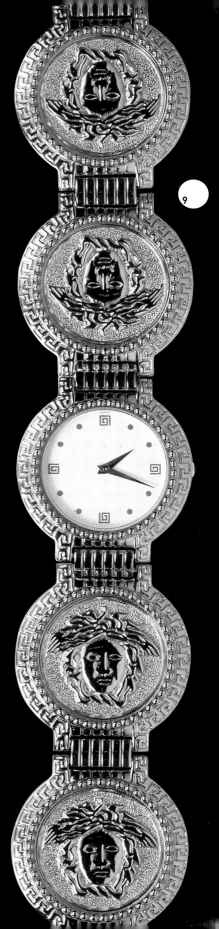

first established itself South of Houston, it would have felt exceptional, but then as a pioneer, not as a survivor. Today, in 2001, there are about 120 galleries in SoHo; five years ago there were more than 200. That was an age in which gallerists, with much the same aspirations as the lords of international fashion, though with rather more attenuated turnovers, understood the specific attractions of the district for the art dealer: its low rents, its sense of being the place, simultaneously cool and hot, its proximity to a vibrant community of artists, its accessibility to collectors. Before the turn of the millennium, gallerists were quickly acknowledging the superior virtues of Chelsea and migrating north and west across Manhattan: more than fifty SoHo galleries, most of them major presences in the art world, relocated there between 1995 and 2000. In 2002 this gallery, too, will relocate, not to Chelsea though but to the meat-packing district around West 13th Street. Like SoHo, Chelsea is already art history.

A decade or more before the galleries arrived en masse in SoHo, the artists had migrated here from Greenwich Village. Sculptors, painters, film-makers, conceptualists, recognized the specific attractions of this former garment-making district, its manufactories upped-and-gone to the lower costs, economies of scale and ease of access on offer in prosaic New Jersey. SoHo had cheap space and no one else was much interested in the area. In 1975 a 3,000-foot SoHo loft could be rented for $450, and even though it felt like a lot of money many young artists took

advantage of the offer. Today a vacant space here will drain $6,000 a month from your account, which is not the kind of cash many artists take home, nor, despite rumours to the contrary, that many gallerists.

SoHo's recent social history highlights the gearing of art's production and sale to the operations of high-end fashion retailers and the property market. That one wave followed another here, each gradually displacing the other, was no isolated instance. In London, since the early 1990s, when young merchant bankers judged inner-city studios more fashionable than Thames-side apartments, a hot-spot of hip has migrated steadily from Clerkenwell to Hoxton and Shoreditch and beyond. The galleries have moved, too – Victoria Miro their highest profile flag-bearer from Cork Street to canal-side – and meantime a diaspora of artists in search of their own myth, the cheap studio, is impelled ever further towards the margins of the city on a rising wave of rents. For a few months at least, in the spring of 2001, Stratford is the new black.

SoHo shifted from art into fashion the way that models slip between one season's garments and the next. The architecture of display remained much the same: what it had borne vanished as attention was diverted by what it carried now. The district underwent a kind of death – its art scene died, at least for its artists – and it went on to experience continual little deaths, those catenating pleasures of extinction and discovery that fashion inflicts upon its victims with every aesthetic convulsion,

every innovation, that is, when we pause for thought, espresso and a cigarette, revealed as no more than an amnesiac restitution of the past.

Varieties of death, however, can exhibit an uncanny sameness. One of the consequences of SoHo's transformation was a convergence of gallery and store. When Helmut Lang planned his Greene Street outlet he chose as architects the New York practice of Gluckman Mayner, who fitted the project in between their existing commitments to relocating art galleries in London and Manhattan. Spaces emerged so minimal, so stripped of merchandise, it was sometimes hard to tell who sold what, if anything, to whom. The confusion was multiplied by the close resemblance of gallery girls to their shop assistant kid sisters and the affection of all for the oeuvres of Helmut Lang and Miuccia Prada. For a while, in the equally perfervid environment of Orchard Street, a few blocks into the Lower East Side, bona fide fashion stores such as Seven put a curator on a salary and maintained exhibition spaces.

These ambivalent domains sometimes erected duplicitous memorials to SoHo's transilience and their own willingness to embrace art. In Comme des Garçons, Silvia Kolbowski and the architect Peter Eisenman built a structure that deliberately hampered access to the store, then installed within it a video which showed simultaneously catwalk footage from the fashion house's newest collection and, its models trailing like disgruntled spectres, the near-forgotten designs of the previous season.

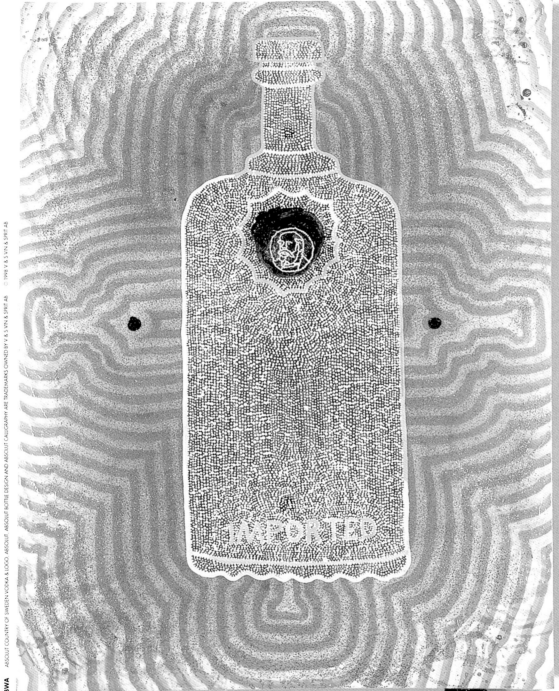

ABSOLUT OFILI.

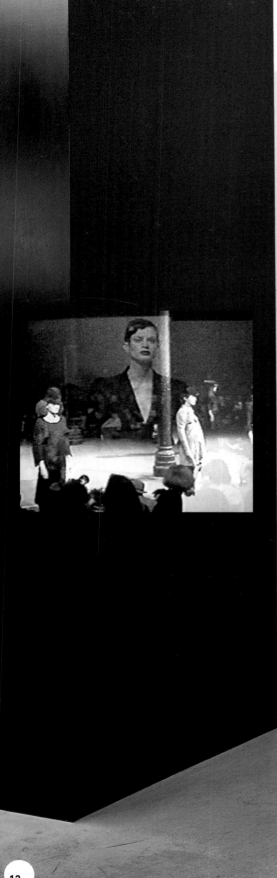

inset
**Silvia Kolbowski
and Peter Eisenman**
*Like the Difference between
Autumn/Winter '94/'95 and
Spring/Summer '95*, 1995,
installed in Comme des Garçons
store, Wooster Street, New York
Videotape frame

So last season: time past meets
time present as the catwalks of
different seasons weave through
each other, models trailing in and
out of each other's bodies like
disgruntled spectres, wearing
the near-forgotten designs of
the previous season.

main picture
Gluckman Mayner Architects
Interior of Helmut Lang store,
New York, completed 1997

opposite
Gluckman Mayner Architects
Interior of Helmut Lang
Parfumerie, New York,
completed 2000

Ambivalent domains: spaces
so stripped of merchandise it
is hard to tell who sells what,
if anything, to whom. The white
cube of exhibition is copied by
the white cube of retailing.
What is on sale, in both, is as
much conceptual as material.

*Like the Difference between Autumn/Winter
'94/'95 and Spring/Summer '95* was, like its
self-consciously obstructive title, hard to
get around. Kolbowski and Eisenman
reflected not only on fashion's willed
occlusions of its immediate past but also
on what had just happened to SoHo as a
district. The deaths were both aesthetic
and geographic, simultaneously separate –
within art, within fashion – and mutual –
the deaths of their collective engagement.
Funded by a fashion designer, Kolbowski
and Eisenman commemorated these
fatalities in a crypt which made their
effacement, their forgetting, blatant.

When I first came to SoHo in the
autumn/winter of '94/'95 the art dealer
Holly Solomon traded from Mercer Street.
Coming to New York to research this book
I'd chosen, for personal and romantic
reasons, to occupy myself in the Chelsea
Hotel rather than the sleeker, model-
draped minimalism of Ian Schrager's
Hudson. I needed to talk to Solomon about
a young artist, Elisa Jimenez, who was
contracted to the gallery and who, evidence
suggested, might be suitable for both the
book and the exhibition I was planning.
Unexpectedly, I found the dealer in a suite
opposite mine on the Chelsea's third floor.
Her gallery had exchanged SoHo's now
exorbitant rents for the faded avant-garde
uncertainties of a hotel that for three
decades had been home to a ferment of
artists, rock musicians and bohemians.
In going there Holly Solomon was making
a statement of some importance. Other,
bigger, galleries had moved out to
expensive, name-architect-designed

spaces further west, where Barbara
Gladstone could be found down the street
from Metro and Paula Cooper in a few tight
blocks rimmed by many of the city's best
restaurants. Collectors, after all, need
entertaining. Solomon, in low-budget, grainy
contrast, had stepped back into art's past,
into one of the few places in New York
where the amphetamine-white wraiths of
the avant-garde still walk, fuelled only by
the purity of their art.

Or perhaps not. When Andy Warhol filmed
his anomic masterwork, *The Chelsea Girls*,
in the hotel many of his acolytes were
ex-fashion models: Nico, Edie Sedgwick,
International Velvet. A former fashion
illustrator of considerable talent and
technique, Warhol was never less than
wholly in thrall to the commodity and to
death, those twinned components of the
modern world that meet and mingle in
fashion. To universal horror, Andy brought it
to everyone's attention that the commodity
and death carried on in much the same way
within art. In their squeak and gibber, the
confidence of the Chelsea's ghosts is that
the engagement of art and fashion didn't
begin in 1990, or 1980, or 1970. Indeed that
last, arbitrary date may be the point of their
furthest separation – as near as we get to
an anti-history. If you silence the spectres
long enough you can almost hear Cecil
Beaton's shutter closing on Jackson
Pollock's paintings, backdrops for a 1951
fashion shoot; almost hear Man Ray, in
1920s Paris, apologetically negotiating
the complex seam of compromise which
allowed his studies of Poiret's dresses,
shot on mannequins for *Vogue*, to appear

in the historically conscious, aesthetically pure pages of that avant-garde organ, *La Révolution surréaliste*. Old friends, art and fashion go back a long way. So far indeed that even at the nascence of modernity, in mid-nineteenth-century Paris, Balzac was taking payments from fashion houses to mention their latest products in his novels. And that is further back than even the longest memory of the Chelsea's inhabitants.

A couple of nights after my arrival, Elisa Jimenez had staged a performance in the Chelsea. Not ghosts, that night, but models, their every step composed, thoughtful, as they processed in Jimenez's sculptural, built-on-the-body clothes. For the marginally more intellectual architecture of this project, Jimenez was also a perfect fit. Neither artist nor fashion designer, both fashion designer and artist, were she not such a confident and motivated individual we might imagine her as confused about the category of creativity to which she belongs. Perhaps she doesn't need to know. Jimenez occupies a category that unsettles and refutes the facile orders that critics decree for culture; a classification as manifold and opalescent as the folded fabric of her dresses. Jimenez retails her individually crafted outfits in select stores in Los Angeles and New York. Some of Hollywood's best-known actresses wear her works. Holly Solomon sells Jimenez's drawings and 'sculptures' to art world collectors, and arranges their loan to art exhibitions throughout the USA. If Elisa Jimenez is both cause and symptom of a category confusion, that ambivalence extended to what I saw in the Chelsea Hotel.

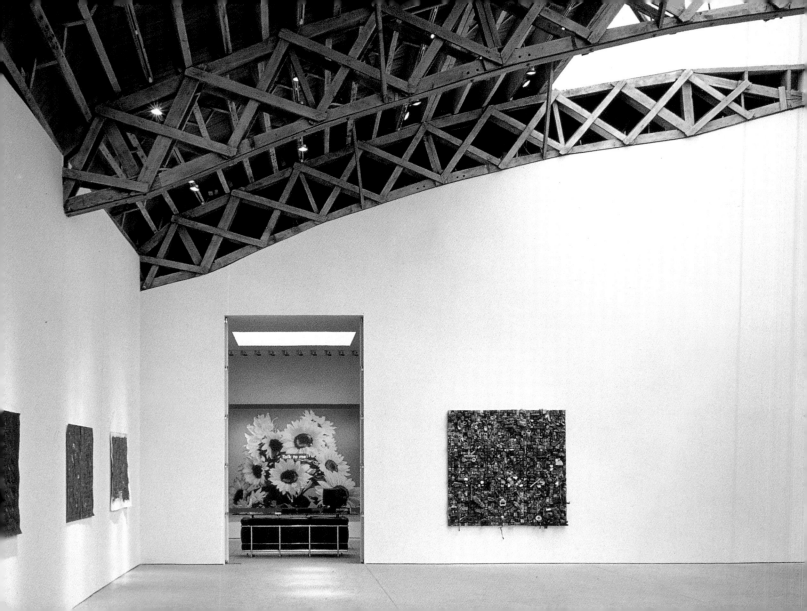

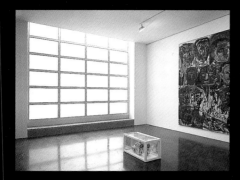 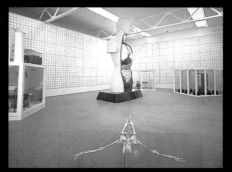

above
Gluckman Mayner Architects
Interior of Gagosian Gallery,
New York

opposite
Gluckman Mayner Architects
Interior of Mary Boone Gallery,
New York

When Helmut Lang exhibits
a Jenny Holzer or Issey Miyake
commissions Frank Gehry to
design a new store, what is the
purpose of that space? Is it still
retail? If so, what is the role of
the artwork, what the role of
architecture?

Was it 'performance' – that loose category
of expressive bodily presence that
emerged in the 1960s – or was it a fashion
show? The models had, after all, worn
objects that would be sold. The staging
commodified Jimenez's creations – just
as their sale through a commercial gallery
would. Art and fashion have the commodity
in common, but until recently perhaps one
party has been rather more reluctant than
the other to admit their shared values.

The dynamics of New York's rent controls
and property market mean that some of
the pioneer artists of the 1970s still
live in SoHo, the trajectories of their
careers arcing upwards along with the
neighbourhood. Working in the wake
of minimalism, theirs was, at first,
a generation in which a terror of the
commodity – of both the object in art and
of their art becoming consumable object –
translated into phobias about fashion. When
fashion was addressed it was, alternately,
in the irreverent performances of Robert
Kushner at Food, fruit substituted for
more durable garments, and the critical
challenges of feminist artists such as
Hannah Wilke to the stereotyping
constraints of costume.

Judith Shea's first important group
exhibition, which took place when she was
still a young artist, was post-minimalism's
apogee – the ground-zero exploration of
PS1 that was 'Rooms', as an abandoned
public school in Queens shifted register to
gallery. Shea's contribution, *King and Queen*,
1976, consisted of two cut and folded blank
canvases, taken down from the stained and

pitted walls for the exhibition's 'prom' as
over-scale ceremonial robes for the guests
of honour. From that moment of almost-
absence, of a near nullification of art's
language and its visuality, Shea would
proceed to reinterpret fashion as a means
of escaping post-minimalism's implosion
of the object. Fashion would be used to
reintroduce first shape, then colour
and finally dimension, all accompanied
by narrative.

A similar trajectory, and a similar complicity
with fashion, albeit manifested in a very
different medium, would be undertaken
by Shea's contemporary, Cindy Sherman.
Even as Sherman demonstrated the
embedding of female stereotypes as the
subject of popular culture in her 'Untitled
Film Stills', she seemed simultaneously to
acknowledge and celebrate the mass media
she pathologized. From the early 1980s,
in a series of collaborations with fashion
designers, Sherman not only revealed her
imbrication as an artist in the processes of
popular culture, but actively participated in
them. By 1993 Sherman would bring her
established cachet as an artist, and her
distinctive look, to the pages of *Harper's
Bazaar*, photographing the spring
collections as if she were a fashion
photographer.

One of those artists who moved to SoHo in
the 1970s, Sherman is still here, living only
a few blocks from the art space where I'm
meditating on Frank Moore's disturbing
imagination. Sherman's loft is across the
street from Kirna Zabête, one of SoHo's
hipper independent stores, and occasionally

Judith Shea
King and Queen, 1976
(photographed in the artist's
studio and worn by Herbert
and Dorothy Vogel)
Canvas

The primary material of art
– the blank canvas – made
simultaneously sculptural
(through the dimensions of
its wearers) and ceremonial
costume. Fashion emerges
from post-minimalism's
implosion of the object.

she crosses it to buy dresses there designed by, amongst others, Elisa Jimenez. That transaction, between artist-as-celebrity and fashion-designer-artist, effected in a chic boutique, is as telling a compression of the current relationship of art and fashion as Moore's painting. In two decades we've seen the emergence of artists who share the mythic media status of Hollywood actresses and fashion models; artists who in their work seamlessly commute between what were once, and in some places still are, imagined as unique and widely separated domains. In the wake of these pioneers has grown up a generation – Elisa Jimenez and contemporaries such as Karen Kimmel – who see these previously distinct fields of practice not so much as having been unified, but as always having been identical.

The formal and story-telling properties embodied within fashion have helped some artists emerge from the apparent dead-end of post-minimalism, but that critique of the aura of the object and language as ideological linchpin has also implicated itself in fashion's reconsideration of its own objectivity. It's hard to imagine that deconstruction of 'fashion as nature' that is an Ann Demeulemeester suit – a garment that reflects on its own 'suitness', its exposed seams evidence of conjunction, its fabric signifying fabrication – without thinking of the gestures of the generation who showed with Judith Shea in PS1, of Gordon Matta-Clark's incisions into architecture, of Michelle Stuart's displacements of one space into another. Perhaps we see in Demeulemeester's work,

or Martin Margiela's, what Jeremy Gilbert-Rolfe has suggested: that fashion performs a role of which art is no longer capable.[1] Where art, informed by critical theory, largely figures only theory's hypostatization, fashion, less rigorous, in its amnesia less encumbered with a prevailing sense of its own significance, still operates through metonym and synecdoche, still allows room for divergent and potentially frivolous readings that celebrate the object even as they reorder it.

Since the mid-1970s, when the handmade glamour of punk aesthetics responded more readily to fashion's technical possibilities than to the austerities of theory, artists have seen fashion as a source of formal solutions and thematic interests at least as often as practitioners within fashion – whether designers, art directors or photographers – have turned to art as a site for stylistic appropriations. Art responds to fashion through fashion's forms; through its anthropologies; through its potential for subjective imagination – our wish, as Karen Kilimnick puts it, to *be* everyone in the fashion magazines. We can simplify the present closeness, that mutuality which encourages fashion houses to advertise in specialist art journals and fashion magazines to run gushing features on the latest painting sensation, as originating in art's need for fashion's glamour and wealth, and fashion's search for intellectual credibility. Such superficialities overlook a particular glamour inherent to the avant-garde (often an inversion of values, whether manifested in mid-nineteenth-century romanticization

of the gypsy or late twentieth-century grunge) which hardly needs fashion to affirm its difference. Suggesting that art wants fashion's money, at this moment in history, is to miss the point that the wealthy and the fashionable, who are, let's face it, usually the same people, have been investing in cutting-edge art since the emergence of an art market. And fashion needing an injection of art's seriousness? I suspect that the avant-garde always gave equally effervescent parties, had as much fun. The gravitas of art is less a necessary catechism for artists than for critics. Despite this, perhaps because of the economic and aesthetic convergence, there are critiques raised that still refuse even the ambivalent positions of Kolbowski and Eisenman, Shea or Sherman. Most of these challenges remain grounded in a resistance to the commodity, coupled with a pathologization of pleasure in looking and being looked at, that would, for our own good, avert our gaze from Medusa's arresting spectacle.

The ubiquitous Gorgon, however, is a figure that perhaps helps us understand the critical phobias that still seek to distinguish, and privilege, art above the commercial domain of fashion. In a brief essay of 1922 Sigmund Freud addressed the psychoanalytic implications of the Medusa myth, remarking that 'the terror of the Medusa is thus a terror of castration that is linked to the sight of something'.[2] For Freud all things Medusine symbolized the female genitals, surrounded by hair, which when glimpsed by the male child offered irrevocable proof of the possibility

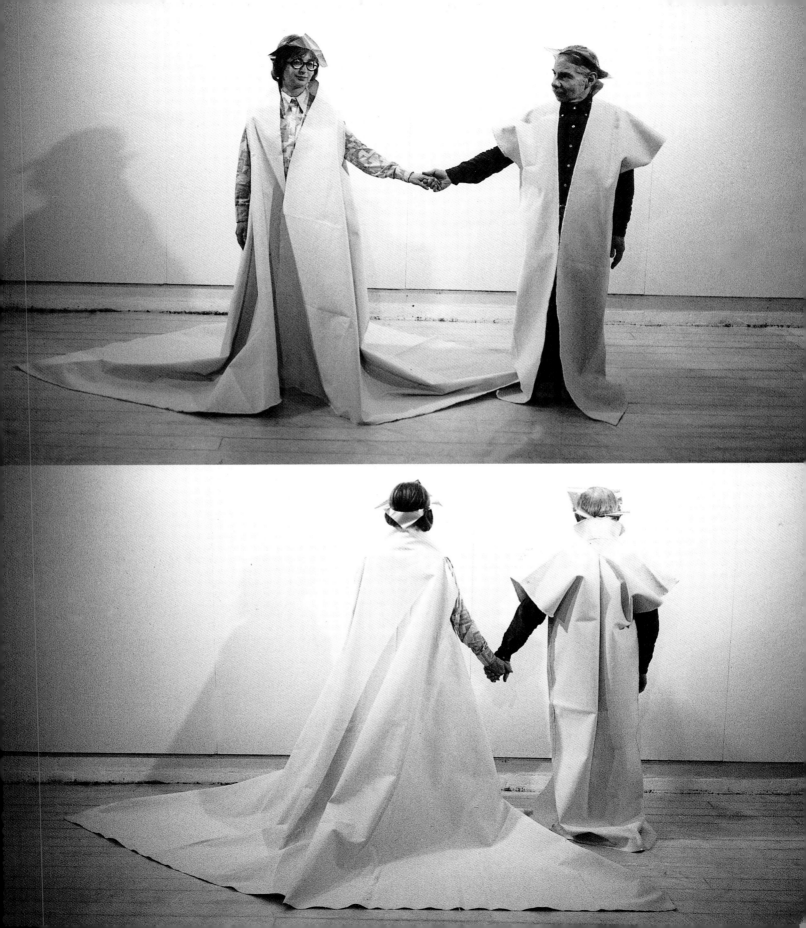

of the loss of his own masculinity. Childish and simplistic as this theory itself is, and without wishing to 'put on the couch' critics who are often all too prepared to put art and artists there, I'd suggest that Frank Moore's representation of Kate Moss as Medusa literalizes a number of fears that permeate critical resistance to fashion and its embrace of art. There is a kind of castration anxiety at work, a dread that this might be what art really looks like behind the veil of representation: disempowered, emasculated. There are two distinctive and often contradictory positions here, and my emphasis on gender in addressing the first of them is not accidental.

Fashion is, within one set of traditional assumptions about culture, largely worn by women and designed by effeminate men. Fashion is crafted from subaltern materials by demeaned, inferior processes such as stitching and sewing. Whereas art, imagined as made with nobler materials, is the pure expression of an individual will in which the hand – and it's usually a male hand – gracefully and immediately answers thought. What I've just caricatured is the discourse by which Renaissance critics and painters refashioned their social status from subordinated artisans to authoritative artists, but it's a discourse that many conservative critics still sustain. Since, at the beginning of this process, elaborate costumes and jewelry were more highly valued than paintings, perhaps an element of the critical phobia towards fashion also begins in the Renaissance. Art is understood to transcend the ephemeral gratification of fashion and offer instead

sustained and weighty meditations on eternal verities. To admit fashion as equivalent is to endanger the discourse by which art established its cultural superiority. It is also to risk the admission that art is, perhaps, less morally valuable, less innately significant, than our traditional ideologies of culture might wish it to be and, equally, rather more inclined towards dangerous, excessive and 'feminine' pleasures.

Beyond the shored defences of gender, the other critical tendency that resists seduction is one for which forms of pleasure are perhaps the greatest problem. At issue here is the purpose of art in culture. Much of the emphasis within this critical mass is directed towards the promotion of art that, literalizing assumptions of a 'psychopathology of the gaze', seeks to substitute for visual pleasure pious reflections on the theoretical, and politically conscious, meanings behind the image. What is seen matters far less than how it is articulated in critical exegesis; the principal satisfaction offered by the image is its ideological challenge to other ideologies. As I've suggested already, with the example of Demeulemeester, fashion is quite capable of wearing a self-critique on its sleeve, but there remain supplementary values peculiar to the object, pleasures of wearing and pleasures of being seen to wear. I'm not so sure that we can discern similar supplementary values in the work of artists engaged in critiques of language and institution – Douglas Huebler, say, or Daniel Buren.

Even in its carefully regulated admission to the institution in the form of major museum shows with curatorial authority, fashion

threatens the ideas that pleasure in general and looking in particular are dangerous deflections from an art whose prime purpose is to reflect on history and – even better – change it. Fashion reminds us that art might belong to some other category of experience than theology. Not only does fashion proceed from an idea that being the object of visual attention is a rather good thing, and that other more corporeal pleasures might derive from this condition; the meanings of its seductive illusions are somewhat slippery phenomena. No friend of the Puritan tendency, the American critic Dave Hickey theorizes the imagery of art as 'sheer, ebullient, slithering, dangerous'.[3] That the look – and, worse, the meaning – of art might be as supple, as fluid, as a dress by Tom Ford for Gucci, circa 1996, and describable in the same terms, are not propositions that academicians and bureaucrats of art are likely to contemplate with equanimity. Despite its frequent avowal of an open-endedness of signification, the critical community within academia insists upon the domestication of art, its subjection to scrutiny and discipline, its explicability. The idea that something might be unfixed, beyond the regulation of categories and their portion-controlled meanings, is profoundly scary. Represented, such an idea might indeed look something like castration, something like death.

Death, of course, is that to which we cannot put an adequate name. In his historical analysis of consumption in nineteenth-century culture, citing Leopardi, Walter Benjamin cried out to fashion, 'Madam Death! Madam Death!'[4] Benjamin was right

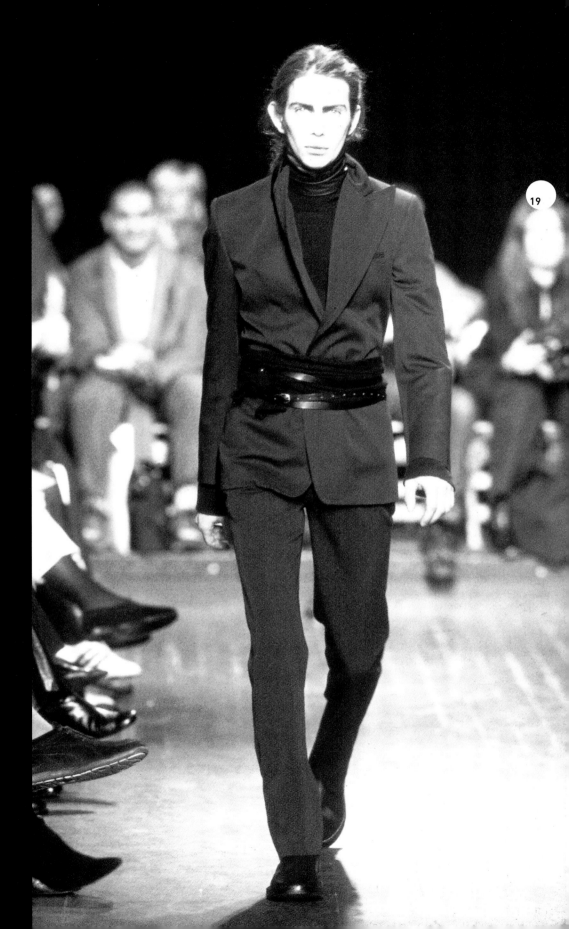

Ann Demeulemeester
Suit, autumn/winter 2001/02

Fashion's own implosion of
the object: a suit that reflects
on its status as suit. Fabric
points out fabrication; exposed
seams highlight conjunction.
Demeulemeester and the other
young Belgian designers make
the same meditations on the
language of their medium as
characterized modernist art.

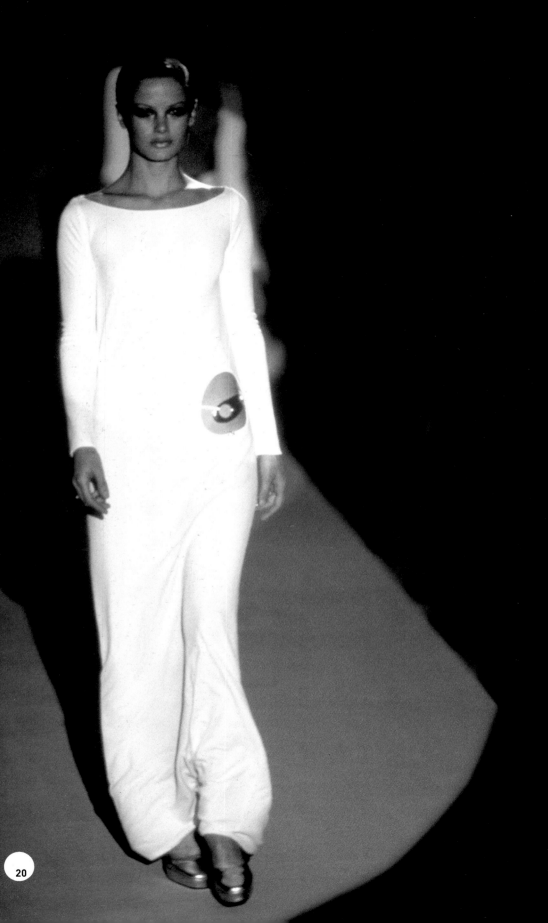

**Gucci
White keyhole dress,
autumn/winter 1996/97**

Is this sensuous and fluid dress,
with its emphasis on visual and
bodily pleasure, both a metaphor
for art's potential meanings and
a model of possible practice?
Is art's embrace of fashion a way
of once more becoming wild, free
and problematic?

but speaking twice still named only half the problem. Frank Moore, bounding his painting with a mirrored frame, allows us to speculate not only on his slaughtered subject but also on our own speculation, our interpolation into that death. The novelist John Barth, in his sequel to the Perseus myth, has a character suggest that, understanding her monstrosity for the first time only in its reflection in the murdering hero's shield, Medusa desired her imminent dispatch.[5] Seeing ourselves see death we contemplate our own monstrosity, an ugliness from which no fashion can ultimately save us. Having proceeded thus far, somewhat like Perseus, by indirection, I want to argue directly here that the mordant pleasures on offer in reflecting on my reflecting on the severed head of a monstrous beauty suggest that the convergences of art and fashion are more than just historical, but also conceptual, and that both historically and conceptually the two are always already converged, endlessly repeating one's gaze at the other. Incidentally, and perhaps more radically, for it demands a reimagining of the sensibility of the entrepreneurial mind to which I'm ill-accustomed, I'd like to think that Gianni Versace understood this when he commissioned *To Die For*.

Death is, supposedly, that at which we never want to look. It is that which, in its ultimate intrusion, destroys meaning. As Kolbowski and Eisenman perceived, in its seasonality the fashion industry turns death over with the rapacity of a medieval graveyard, periodically returning to examine and sometimes resurrect the corpses that this

rotation exhumes. Medusa is, as Jacques Lacan observed in his analysis of Freudian theory, that 'which properly speaking is unnameable ... the image of death in which everything comes to its end'.[6] Medusa also signifies for Lacan the presence of the Real, that condition which destroys both the symbolic register of language that orders our lives and the imaginary register of our subjective relationship to the world. Lacan wrote of the Real as 'the essential object which isn't an object any longer, but this something with which all words cease and all categories fail, the object of anxiety *par excellence*'.[7] Lacan was describing a philosophical and psychological category of experience, but he might as well have been talking about fashion, or Medusa its fearful exemplar. With fashion, the essentiality of any object – its reason for existence – is ceded with each season. The object no longer is. And in ceasing, in being first something to die for and then nothing, for which you died – without your ever receiving the satisfaction, the truth, that it promised – fashion works as an object of anxiety. Which is perhaps why we like it so much.

It's here, in failure, that art critics discover their greatest fear of art. What if, like fashion, art doesn't mean enough? And it seems to me that, beyond the commercial transactions, the shared social circles, the exchange of intellectual status with glamour and wealth, and even the redistribution of aesthetic ideas, this is where art and fashion have always met, now in 2001 as in 1921 or 1851. What both promise and both fail to deliver is the

satisfaction of ultimate meaning. Of course, fashion and art are not unique in this failure of meaning – a level at which anything means nothing, signifies only death – but few other objects of desire in our culture promise quite so fervently that they, uniquely, are the ones with the answer you seek. Few other objects are quite so heartbreaking in the ways in which they inflict their disappointments. Their significations, when you reach out for them, are empty and you are left to fall back on resources of self-identity wholly depleted by your desire. What you get in recompense is pleasure, which is what you hope will be the assuaging of desire, but which always turns out to be a near-miss. Art as much as fashion is inadequate, its promises of profundity and historical effectiveness chimeric, the circularity of its history a perpetual slipping away from delivering the punch line at the appropriate moment. Art and fashion: you always need more, or you settle for nothing. But rather than despair, our response here should perhaps be one of relief. What if art, any more than fashion, *could* offer us an ultimate truth? What would we do after the end of art? ●

New York, April 2001

1

CONCEPTUALISM AND FASHION'S REJECTION

IN DRESSING ONE CREATES AN IMAGE: AN IMAGE TO BE READ

Antony McCall and Andrew Tyndall
Argument, 1978

Victor Burgin
Lei-feng, 1973–4
One of nine photographic panels:
photograph on paper

Fashion exposed in an analysis
of how signs convince us of their
naturalness. Burgin's disjunction
of picture and text forces us to
re-examine the content of an
image that seems wholly normal,
whilst simultaneously concealing
its own agenda.

Smiling, a young woman looks away from the sheaf of magazines that lie beside her on a fur coat. Her blonde hair is woven into coiled plaits; she wears a flower-printed dress with a high waistline and narrow collar. The girl might be the focus of a painting, a suitable subject for Vermeer, but she is in fact the subject of firstly an advertisement and secondly an artwork, *Lei-feng,* 1973–4, by the British photographer Victor Burgin. The girl is crowded with relations – immediate ones such as family, for two older characters, who are 'read' as her mother and father, are also in the picture, and it is they at whom she smiles, they who engage with each other through an exchange of looks at their daughter. More distanced are the picture's other 'relations' – a certain resonance between the girl's dress and the foliage of a garden half-seen through the lights of a bay window. If this line of signification is consciously constructed to represent the girl as 'natural', it is complemented and modified by the vase of flowers at the right edge of the picture, the fur behind it, and the floral pattern of the table on which the vase rests. The girl is nature brought inside, acculturated.

What that culture might be is reflected in a proliferation of the girl's face – the fashion magazine cover as tangential mirror. This is not a 'real' *Vogue* cover, of course. The advertisers have used the magazine's status as bearer of iconic fashion, its signification of sophistication, in a more complex construction of values. The girl has just appeared on the cover of *Vogue* – perhaps for the first time – and her parents share their joy in her success. What do this trio of sophisticates choose for their celebration? A bottle of blended, proprietary sherry.

The advertisement tells us a great deal: about the values which the manufacturers and marketeers wanted to convey about their product, about the incidental values and status of family life and visual beauty in the early 1970s when the advertisement was made, and about the relationship of artists to popular culture and the consumer society at that time. As an artwork the picture tells only half the story. Victor Burgin 'took' this picture, appropriating it rather than making it as a photograph. It's unlikely that Burgin would have bothered with the lumbering, blatant composition or the picture's carefully manipulated lighting. The constructed nature of the advertising image is Burgin's subject in *Lei-feng,* and he makes it apparent by juxtaposing the same picture across nine panels with different textual accompaniments. These texts do not analyse the picture, though at other times Burgin and his contemporaries did decode advertisements rather than describe *how* they communicated. The texts are detailed theorizations of semiotic systems – statements about how signs work. *Lei-feng* is concerned with the underlying ideological structures of pictures, even of innocent sherry advertisements; structures which efface themselves to make the message they bear appear as natural as the leaves brushing the windows of a suburban villa.

The disconnection of picture and image, however, has another effect. This too is ideological, and in countering an ideology that presupposes family relations, beauty, bourgeois comfort and blended sherry as naturally good things, it too occludes its intention, this time through the distraction of radical juxtaposition rather than the coherence of pictorial representation. What emerges in the fissure between image and text is a critique of the commodity, of the culture of capitalist production and the social relations which that economic system implies. The pleasure, the surplus, of bourgeois life – whether sherry, cut flowers or fashionable dresses and furs – is achieved at the expense of someone else's (hidden) exploitation.

In the 1970s, revealing the interpolation of fashion into this system of commodity relationships, and providing a counter-critique, were urgent concerns for an increasingly radical and politically motivated body of artists. Where, in the 1960s, fashion had often been intimate with art, whether, for example, in Warhol's oeuvre or in the stylistic correspondences between Lucio Fontana as artist and Bini-Telese as designer, the subsequent decade witnessed a withdrawal by artists from what were increasingly understood as the corrupting pleasures of commodity culture. Fashion functioned as a moral index for the perceived inadequacies of an economic system. Fashion represented one element of what Marxist critics called 'false consciousness' – the misrecognition of the real conditions of existence, one's subordination and exploitation, through investments in the lure of particular commodities. Fashion, repeatedly invoking freedom in its advertising, promises a transformation of the self, or a realization of the true self, that in reality not only depends upon the continued subordination of the individual – for you must work, be exploited, in order to buy the commodity – but upon the subordination of others who are exploited to produce the object of desire.

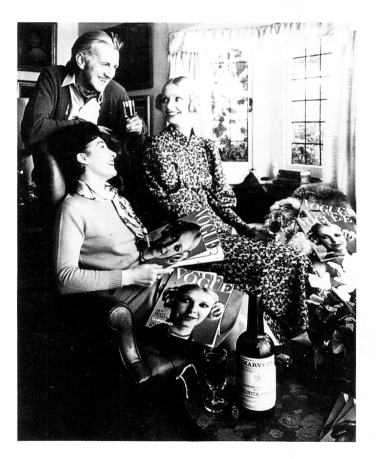

Together they study the texts through which they may improve their ideological formation.

Martinent has criticised Hjelmslev's treatment of *expression* and *content* as logically discrete domains, "...one speaks to be understood," he says, "and the expression is at the service of the content." In Hjelmslev's scheme the expression purport of speech is the range of humanly producible sounds. These are the object of the science of *phonetics* and the forms which languages impose upon this common purport are described in the science of *phonology*. Martinet observes that there is no science which bears the relation to Hjelmslev's content-purport that phonology bears to phonetics. He moreover doubts that such a science is theoretically feasible as its descriptions, being symbolically expressed, would necessarily be cast in accordance with prior articulations of content. "There is," he says, "no para-linguistic discipline...which would enable us to handle a psychic reality prior to any integration into linguistic frameworks."

The significance to semiotics of such observations has been stated by Todorov, semiotics "...will never be dealing with anything other than linguistic signification, surreptitiously substituted for the real object. Semiotics of the non-linguistic area is short-circuited, not at the level of its object (which undoubtedly exists), but at that of its discourse which infiltrates the verbal into the results of its work."

Hjelmslev conceived of semiology as a meta-semiotic investigation which would locate the irreducible differences between signifying systems, thus establishing a semiotic typology. Within this typology we might place a semiotics of photography. At the technical level such a semiotics would aim to describe the range of actual and potential codes of photographic reproduction. These codes would then be considered in their functions as frameworks for world-views. At this stage the verbal will indeed have fully infiltrated the work. It is to be accepted that semiotics, albeit informed by, incorporating, and transforming models from the exact sciences, cannot give an 'ontologically pure' account of its object - of the "rhetoric of the image." Todorov rightly observes that "semiotics is for the moment still a system of propositions rather than a body of established knowledge." In this recognition we may therefore opt for a theoretically self-conscious intervention in the production of photographic rhetoric, for a 'critical practice' where semiotics, ideology and aesthetics meet.

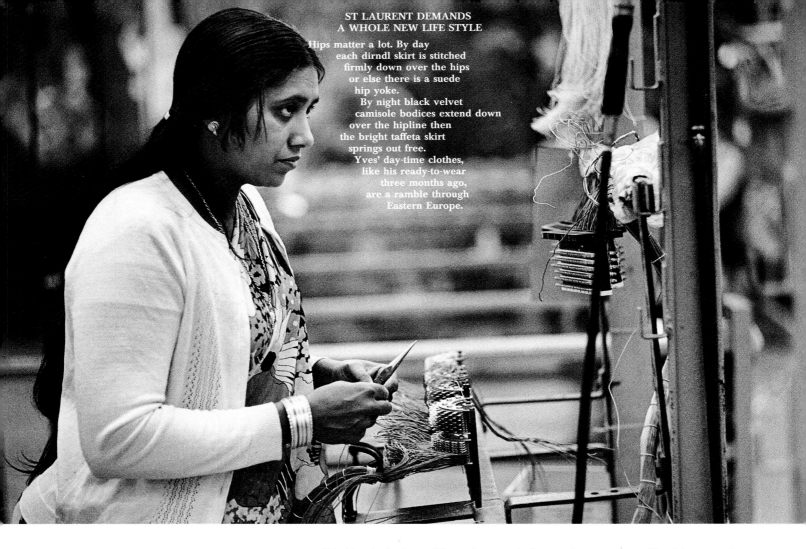

ST LAURENT DEMANDS
A WHOLE NEW LIFE STYLE

Hips matter a lot. By day
each dirndl skirt is stitched
firmly down over the hips
or else there is a suede
hip yoke.
By night black velvet
camisole bodices extend down
over the hipline then
the bright taffeta skirt
springs out free.
Yves' day-time clothes,
like his ready-to-wear
three months ago,
are a ramble through
Eastern Europe.

If fashion, in the form of *Vogue*, is a marginal but telling element within *Lei-feng*, it becomes a vital issue in Burgin's series 'UK, 76'. *St Laurent demands a whole new life style*, 1976, appropriates the text of a fashion magazine, describing garments from a new collection that abstracted racial otherness and made it exotic. There is only description, no illustration of this hyperbolized, romanticized peasant or gypsy look. Instead Burgin depicts an Indian woman in a cardigan and brightly printed sari, concentrating on her task of industrial production. Where *Lei-feng* worked through apparent disjunction, *St Laurent demands...* establishes significant connections between image and text that promote and efface a particular ideology – that of the critique of commodity relations – rather than analyzing how ideology works. Perhaps the most significant of these connections is a direct physical relation between the worker and the text. The left edge of the description

conforms to the profile of the woman's forehead. This is supplemented by the woman's ethnicity: she is not obviously 'read' as Indian, but through skin colour, costume and jewelry is understood as exotic and oriental. She might be one of the Romanies or peasant Slavs romantically imagined by Yves Saint Laurent.

In her hand the woman holds a pair of scissors. Before her is a piece of equipment on which there are plaited fibres and bobbins. The device looks like a spinning machine. Again a connection is made. Is this one of the exoticized peasants paradoxically working in a sweat shop to produce if not the very garments that parody the real conditions of her existence, then something very like them? The obviousness of photographs encourages their rapid scrutiny, a degradation of attention. The ideological programme of Burgin's picture utilizes this facility. Those are not scissors the woman

Victor Burgin
*St Laurent demands a
whole new life style,* 1976,
from the series 'UK, 76'
Photographic panel

Contrasting the fantasy invoked
by fashion's imagination of the
world as it should be – but
never can be – with the life-
numbing realities of the world
as it is, including the industrial
production of fashion and its
fantasies.

holds, they are electrical pliers. She is not
weaving fibres but fine electrical cables,
engaged in the complex and skilled task of
assembling what might be the wiring loom of
a car. Burgin equates this labour with that of
an exploited seamstress so that all forms of
industrial labour appear equally demeaning
and exploitative, and suggests that fashion
plays a significant role in such exploitation.

By the mid-1970s fashion's effect upon
the individual had also become a familiar
subject for feminist artists. Fashion was
understood as a masculine construct
through which women were accustomed
to fitting subordinate, gendered social
roles and which imposed particular physical
demands upon the female body. Influenced
by Brechtian aesthetics and, like Burgin,
convinced of the imperative that art's primary
task was an overtly ideological education
of its audience, the American artist Martha
Rosler exemplified mid-'70s feminist

practice. Recycling images from popular
culture, Rosler sought to expose their
hidden ideological premises in much the
same manner as Burgin. The collages of
the 'Body Beautiful' series, begun in 1965,
change the contextual setting of the female
body, encouraging the spectator, as
Alexander Alberro writes, 'to reconsider
the use of women as signs for domesticity,
docility, sexuality and the circulation of
commodities.'[1] Rosler's work concentrates
on making explicit the sexuality that fashion
simultaneously conceals and emphasizes
both as a corporeal trait and as a condition
of identity. It locates woman at the centre
of a visual regime in which the object both
substitutes for her sexuality and, seemingly,
compels it upon her.

Rosler's friend Eleanor Antin placed a
greater emphasis upon autobiography within
her work, establishing herself as a generic
figure for all women, or inhabiting invented

personae. Identity was embedded in, and
emerged from, narrative, whether embodied
in installations or mediated through textual
fictions. Antin's installations assembled
their subjects through consumer products
and household goods. Identity was
conditioned by consumption. This extension
of Pop art strategies contrasted with an
increasingly dominant minimalist aesthetic,
but it also strove to demonstrate the
determination of the female subject by
external, object-based influences. The early
video *Representational Painting*, 1971, is a
droll critique of normative conceptions of
feminine beauty in which Antin transforms
her face from 'ordinary' to 'attractive' with
make-up. As Howard N. Fox notes, 'The
work captures the irony in making arbitrary
distinctions between plain and beautiful,
and it slyly begs the question of why women
subject themselves to this exercise of
making their appearance conform to
preferred tastes.'[2]

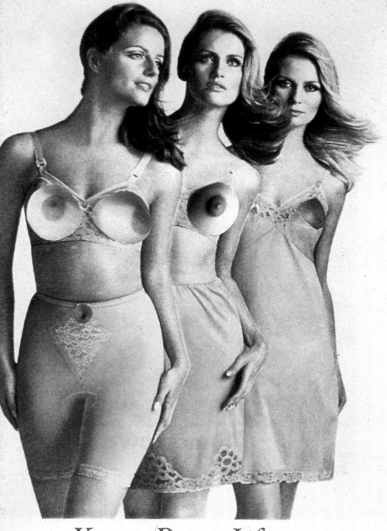

Kayser/Perma-Lift

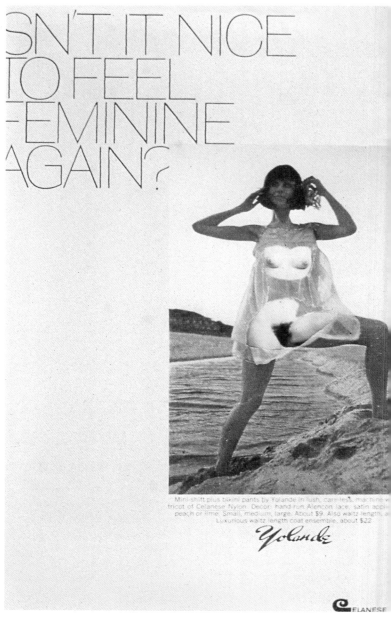

ISN'T IT NICE
TO FEEL
FEMININE
AGAIN?

Martha Rosler
Untitled (S, M, L or Kayser/Perma-Lift), 1972, from the series 'Body Beautiful' (aka 'Beauty Knows No Pain')
Photomontage printed as colour photograph

Collaging purloined imagery from the materials that promote fashion and stereotypes of femininity, Rosler exposes the presuppositions contained within advertising. Fashion becomes the target of an art that itself has a clear ideological purpose.

Martha Rosler
Untitled (Isn't it nice to feel feminine again?), 1967–72, from the series 'Body Beautiful' (aka 'Beauty Knows No Pain')
Photomontage printed as colour photograph

Making explicit the sexuality that fashion simultaneously conceals and emphasizes, Rosler highlights the positioning of the woman's body at the centre of a visual regime that seems to compel sexuality upon her.

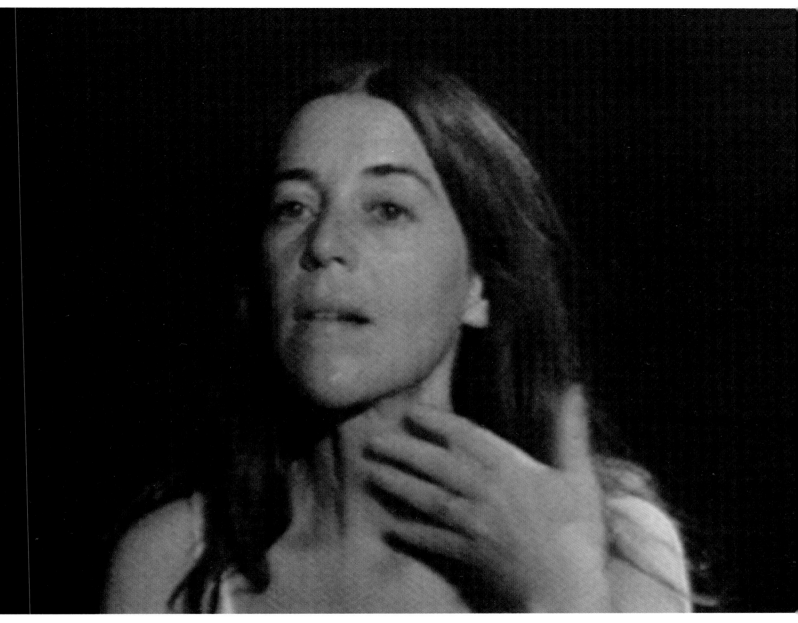

Eleanor Antin
Representational Painting, 1971
Video

A work that, in its duration,
wittily captures the arbitrary
distinctions that distinguish
ordinary from beautiful, and
begs the question as to why
women choose to conform
to particular standards.

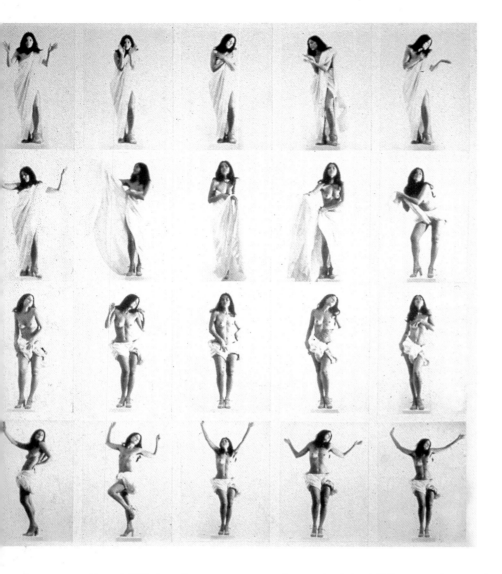

left
Hannah Wilke
Super-T-Art,
Performalist Self-Portrait
with Christopher Giercke, 1974
20 b/w photographs

A self-conscious play with the
most primal vectors of fashion –
one body, one piece of fabric –
which transforms identity as it
goes. Wilke seems to ask, 'Where
is the real me in all of this?'

opposite
Helmut Newton
Office Love
Vogue Hommes, 1976

A social and sexual positioning
of women wholly abhorrent to
radicals and feminists alike,
Newton's work for fashion
magazines seemed to confirm
artists' worst fears about
fashion's promotion of sexual
subordination and passivity.

Hannah Wilke's performances were most often undertaken before a camera rather than an audience. Wilke was sometimes vilified by other feminists for an oeuvre which made a spectacle of her body and created complex explorations of the dynamics of misogyny and women's complicity with their own objectification. In *Super-T-Art*, 1974, Wilke took a piece of fabric and a woman's body – the determining vectors of fashion at their most primal. In a series of photographs the artist disported herself and the fabric, transforming identities as she went. The cloth emphasized as often as it concealed, Wilke flitting from being one *thing* to another. Here Wilke challenged the dominant ideology of 1970s feminism – the notion of an essential identity figured through the female body. Even stripped down to this, the most

basic 'me', Wilke seemed to say, there is no 'woman' here, but rather one made by others and by the imagination of one's 'self'. Wilke represents the initial rethinking of the feminine within feminism and illustrates the role of fashion in self-fashioning. Her grid of images – that distinctively minimalist strategy – opened out the subjective possibilities of the object, rather than foreclosed them.

Fashion's own self-conscious positioning against art through much of the 1970s had to do with minimalism's draining of colour, pattern and form from visual culture. Eventually the formal strategies of minimalism (Calvin Klein et al, 1997) and *arte povera* (Marc Jacobs and the first grunge designers) would find their way into fashion,

but their legitimation was still distant. For much of the decade fashion was going somewhere other than towards art, and that somewhere was often a self-indulgent, nostalgic and orientalizing aesthetic. Within fashion photography, however, there were points of correspondence which presaged a renewed engagement between presently divergent creative practices. Many of Deborah Turbeville's contemporaries were content to reiterate the visual strategies of the 1960s, or else to look back through hazy, Vaseline-smeared lenses to a Golden Age located somewhere between Victoriana and the Jazz Age. By contrast Turbeville's often disquieting imagery seemed to reference the darker aspects of Surrealism – especially the work of Hans Bellmer – and to parallel the problematic of bodily presence that was being examined by some contemporary artists. The highest profile photographers, however, were often working in a medium – colour film – that was antithetical to the monochrome subtleties of contemporary art-photographers as diverse as Duane Michals, Larry Clark and Ansel Adams. Furthermore, the work of Helmut Newton and Guy Bourdin in particular articulated a social and sexual positioning of women that was wholly abhorrent to radical and feminist artists, and that seemed to confirm all of those artists' worst suspicions about fashion as an agency that promulgated subordination and passivity.

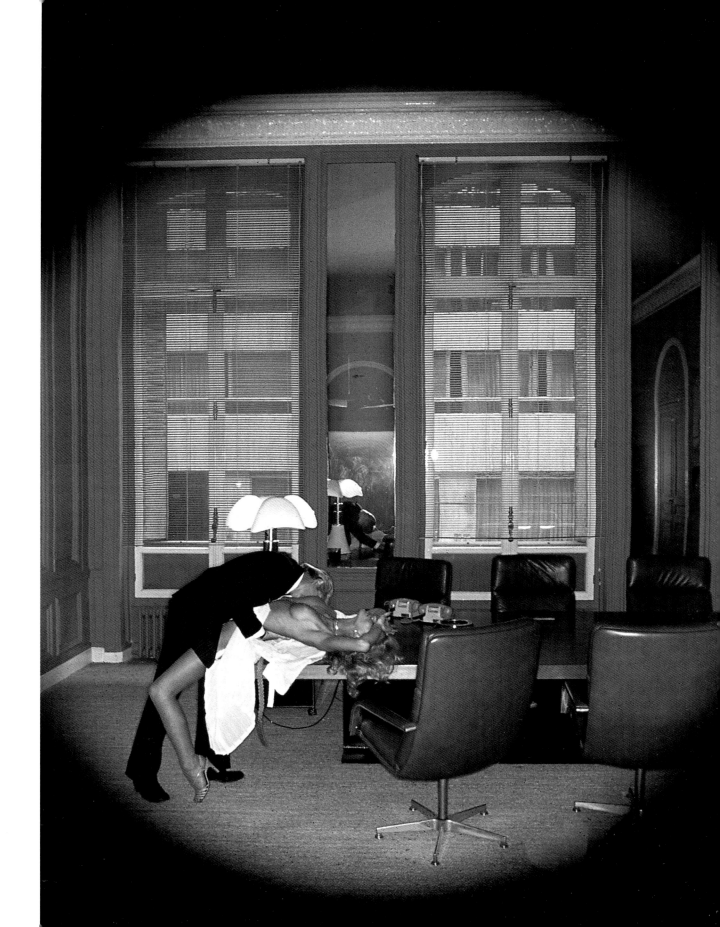

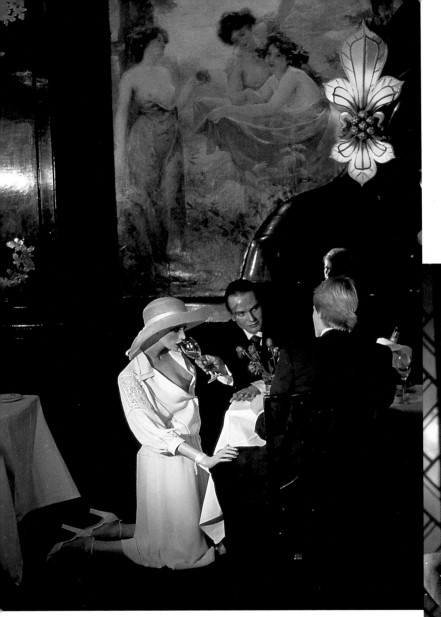

below
Helmut Newton
Store Dummies 1,
French *Vogue*, 1976

In the midst of misogyny,
Newton offers a subversive
alternative in the pages of
a women's magazine. Here
the exchange is between
women, or between a woman
and her mannequin double.
In a solipsism simultaneously
narcissistic and sexual, men
are conspicuously absent.

opposite
Helmut Newton
Maxim's 1,
French *Vogue*, 1978

For a younger generation
of artists and critics, more
concerned with individual
identity than collective action,
Newton seemed to represent
a potential liberation through
sexual transgression and a
refusal of the pastoralization
of sexuality which 1970s
radicalism seemed to promote.

above
Helmut Newton
From the Story of Ohhh,
American *Vogue*, 1975

This image encapsulates how
most feminists understood
Newton's work: the woman is
on her knees, a servile accessory
to a transaction between men.
Is she the object of this exchange,
and are the expensive clothes she
wears nothing more than a token
of their power over her?

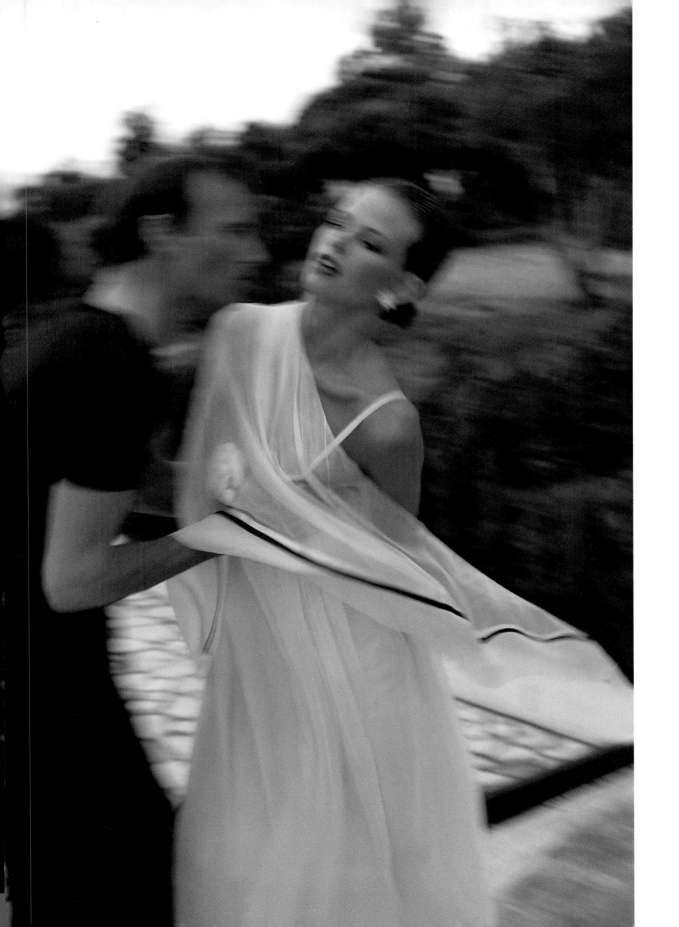

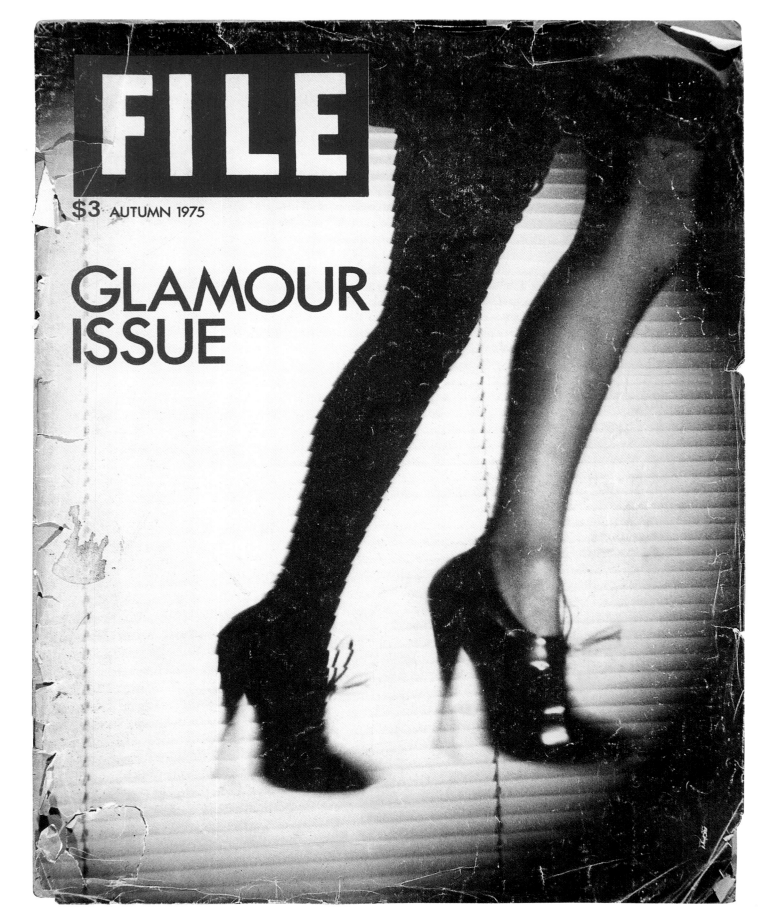

FILE

$3 AUTUMN 1975

GLAMOUR ISSUE

General Idea
File magazine cover,
autumn 1975

Inspired by William Burroughs
('language is a virus') and
Marshall MacLuhan ('the medium
is the message'), with *File*,
General Idea reconceived both
the art journal and the fashion
magazine, and reconfigured the
relationship of art to life.

General Idea
File magazine spread,
autumn 1975

An ironic appropriation of mass
culture. Using a strategy that
would become common in the
punk era, General Idea subverted
fashion and sent its modified
appearance back as a virus that
would infect fashion for the next
twenty-five years.

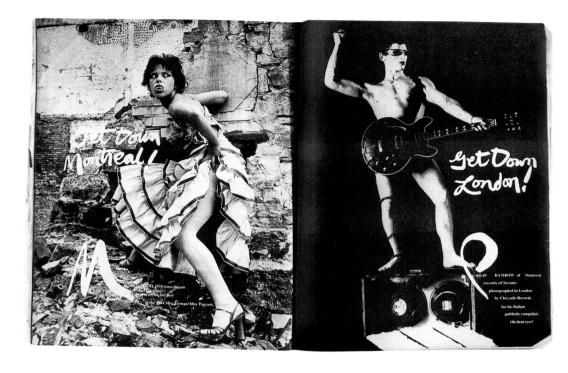

The preface to Newton's 1978 collection, *Sleepless Nights*, went so far as to align the feminist condemnations of the photographer in his defence. 'Looking through these pictures, what does one see? The answer is one's own secret thoughts, dreams and longings.... We are all, on occasion, voyeurs, sadists, freaks – we treat women as objects, if only because we constantly seek to freeze them, as Newton does, in their impossible beauty – like Newton, we think unthinkable thoughts most of the time.'[3] Art, for most of the 1970s, could not entertain the unthinkable and sought to redeem thought. Fashion found the unthinkable entertaining.

One of the most succinct encapsulations of Newton's oeuvre came from the critic Rosetta Brooks. 'Clothes to be raped in, shoes to be found dead in, a scarf to be strangled by, the promises of Newton's photographs are of violence, bestiality and death.'[4] Brooks's remark, however, was not contained within a feminist onslaught on misogynistic values. The essay was a studied appraisal of sado-masochistic fashion and the potentially liberating effects of sexual transgression for the individual. Furthermore, Brooks was writing in a radical art magazine, *ZG*, which she edited. For an emerging generation of

artists and critics, Newton had moved from being a pariah to becoming an object of legitimate critical enquiry as well as a stylistic influence. Together with the equally denigrated Guy Bourdin – as well as the older models of Louise Dahl-Wolfe and Cecil Beaton – Newton would have an important effect upon the young Nan Goldin in her switch to colour photography in the mid-1970s, and would exemplify the imaginary decadence which many in her generation would both come to crave, and themselves exemplify, in the next decade.

Newton's own dystopian vision was recognized in *ZG* as a challenge to the 'perfect world' promoted by most advertising, and by fashion magazines. Brooks wrote, 'In the place of sexual harmony and stability, Newton's images were those of conflict and fragmentation. Veiled eroticism became explicit sexuality. The semi-nude made respectable by the paradises of deodorant ads, became threats of the implosion into the hell of city life.'[5] If stylistically conservative, Newton was being considered in critical terms that were still novel for the appraisal of artworks (Brooks invoked Lacan and his concept of the image as trap for the gaze; elsewhere in the magazine Georges Bataille

35

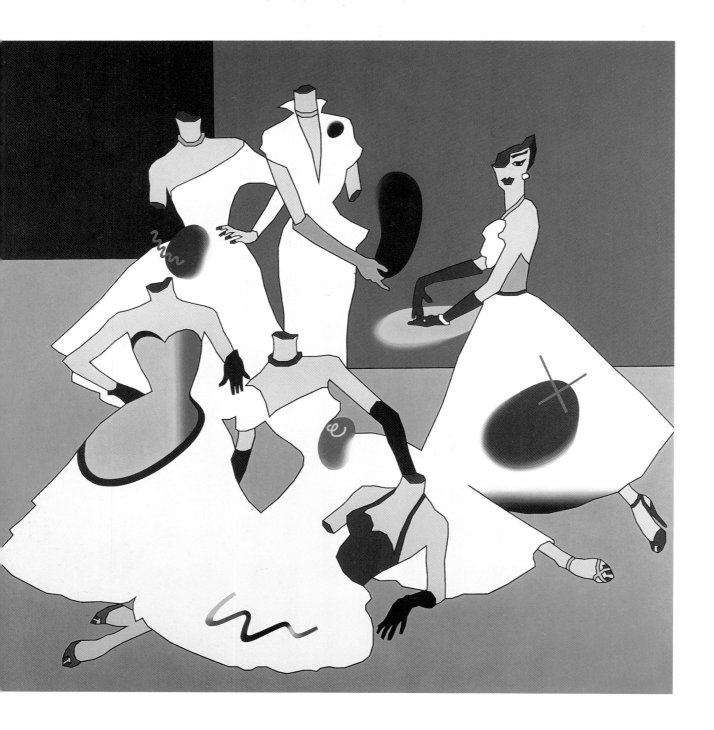

Duggie Fields
Modes of Perception, 1976
Acrylic on canvas

Generations clash: poses and
fashions that invoke the seductive
glamour of the 1950s fashion
plate, subjected to a meditated
and erotic violence against the
figure that might have come from
a Helmut Newton photograph.

Duggie Fields
*Just a Chance Encounter
and Goodness Knows What
Complications May Follow,* 1980
Acrylic on canvas

Painting that in its use of colour,
figure and erotic, languorous
pose – all borrowed from fashion
– challenges the academic
sterility of 1970s British art.

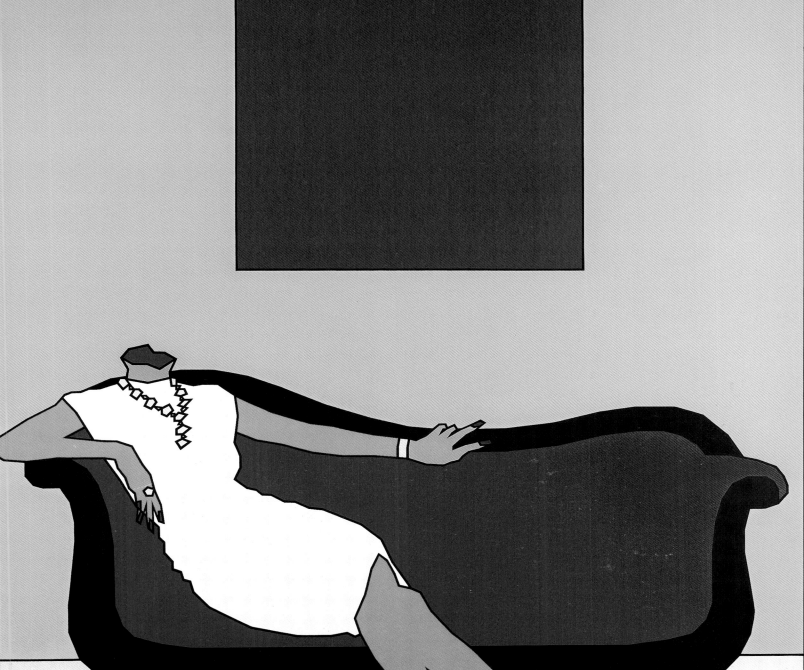

was a dominant influence). Through his use of narrative and the provision of visual pleasure, Newton was understood to be offering models of sexual and psychic excess that were potentially emancipatory. Brooks's article was contained in a special issue of *ZG* which dealt with a wide range of cultural manifestations of S/M and included polemics by lesbian and gay activists Pat Califia and Guy Hocquenghem, an essay on the photographer Jean-Marc Prouveur and an interview with Vivienne Westwood.

Westwood's presence in *ZG* signalled where the magazine was coming from, but simultaneously gave an indication of where cultural critiques would be going in the 1980s. *ZG* emerged from a group of young artists and critics drawn into the London punk scene on the cusp of its transformation into New Romanticism. This hybridized and self-consciously transgressive milieu spawned a magazine that recognized no contradictions in addressing all aspects of culture, including art, music, fashion, film and television, as interconnected. For a generation which had, for a few short years, expressed its identity partly through provocations towards

vestimentary norms, and which, like no youth culture before it, offered a certain emancipation to marginalized sexual identities, accepting the political importance of fashion was not a problem. Its historical relevance was a part of their – to be personal for a moment, our – lived experience. Furthermore, unlike other art magazines of the time, *ZG* offered a theoretical emphasis which both reflected and challenged new academic interests. Brooks's first editorial overtly confronted cultural fragmentation and the critical derogation of popular culture.

This embrace of the popular was exemplified by *ZG*'s first interviewee, the British painter Duggie Fields. Fields didn't look like an artist – least of all a British artist. His studiously cultivated appearance took its reference points from the Edwardian dandy, the mod and a Dalí-esque Surrealism. Fields's similarly citational paintings didn't much look as though they belonged to either established or institutionally approved British art in the mid-1970s. Like punk and New Romantic culture in general, Fields was a provocation to academic sterility and conceptual aridity. That challenge was articulated through colour, eroticism and figural narrative –

all recovered from the imagery and imagination of popular culture. Inspired by the work of the Canadian collective General Idea and their early, ironic attention to fashion, typified by the 1975 'glamour' issue of their magazine *File*, Fields and other British artists of the late 1970s found a 'political' direction for their work. As Fields puts it, 'Glamour replaced Marxism as the revolutionary style statement of the 20th century.'[6]

As Brooks described them, Fields's paintings 'seem to be about the point at which style is dissolving into the symbolic mix of everyday life; the point at which styles merge into the artificiality of our surroundings. They seem to derive their sources not so much from the artists whom Fields quotes, but from the point at which these sources are, in conventional terms, debased by mechanical reproduction/mass production...'[7] A similar strategy, at much the same time, though more overtly informed by a critique of its sources, was being undertaken by Cindy Sherman with her 'Untitled Film Stills' series. Fields shifted the medium from photography to painting, and his highly coloured, large-scale canvases remained closely linked to the compositional tenets and seductive glamour of the classical fashion plate. If this evoked Beaton or Henry Clarke, however, in the fragmentation of his subjects – beheaded ball-gowned models lounging together or alone in works such as *Modes of Perception*, 1976, or *Just a Chance Encounter and Goodness Knows What Complications May Follow*, 1980, the dismembered male torsos of *In Limbo Like Me (Invitation to the Dance)*, 1977 – Fields exercised a meditated and erotic violence against the figure. He invokes the maligned Helmut Newton even as he more overtly cites Pollock, Miró and Mondrian.

General Idea's own agenda within *File*'s 'glamour' issue was expressed in a playful manifesto: 'We knew Glamour was not an object, not an action, not an idea. We knew Glamour never emerged from the "nature" of things. There are no glamorous people, no glamorous events. We knew glamour was artificial. We knew that in order to be glamorous we had to become plagiarists, intellectual parasites.' Against the direct opposition to consumer culture and its values represented by Burgin, Rosler and others, General Idea recognized both their own involvement in the culture they were

attempting to critique and the impossibility of getting 'outside' it to establish some kind of 'truth', some kind of pure point of opposition to a dominant ideology where one was not, in turn, proffering a new set of dominant ideas. Instead the collective used a wholesale, profoundly ironic embrace of the inauthentic as a challenge to the 'authentic' values that were continually presented to them through the mass media.

A. A. Bronson, the surviving member of General Idea, remarks that their strategy in confronting the values purveyed by advertising was to use the same techniques. Inspired by Situationist theory, by William Burroughs's ideas of language as a virus and, perhaps in a more general way, enthused by Marshall MacLuhan's concepts of immediacy and dissemination in the mass media, the trio of Bronson, Felix Partz and Jorge Zontal took the everyday presentations of identity, belief and value that were submitted to them, and returned them to a world with a zesty twist (a twist that was almost literal in 1981's 'Test Tube cocktail'). *File* overtly parodied mass-circulation magazines in both its layout and its title (rearranging *Life*) – and was in turn quickly parodied. Bronson comments that

Andy Warhol's celebrity magazine, *Interview*, switched to colour immediately after Bronson had passed an issue of *File* to Warhol in person, hoping for precisely this effect.

General Idea's strategic placement of art within culture, rather than simply using it as a tool in an ideological conflict, anticipates a wider sharing of values. Though, as conceptual artists, General Idea left few art objects in their wake, their work moves beyond the phobia of the object in both art and culture that is expressed in much avant-garde art of the 1970s. In their concerns, both General Idea and Duggie Fields, in different media, seem to anticipate a convergence, even as fashion is vilified elsewhere in fine art. Motivated by General Idea's interventions, artists such as Fields and Cindy Sherman – who would trek from her college in Buffalo to Toronto to see the collective's work – represented a way forward in the 1980s by opening out narrative spaces, by introducing colour, figuration and even the erotic. Theirs are images that, like Newton's, 'trap the gaze', even as they contest its primacy, and the principal influences upon their development are drawn not from other artists or theoretical debates about art, but from fashion and popular culture ●

2

AMBIVALENT EMBRACE

IF ALL STYLISTS ARE ARTISTS AND ALL ARTISTS HAVE STYLE, A COLLABORATION BETWEEN THE TWO ... SEEM[S] LIKE A GOOD IDEA

The Face
October 1984

Dianne Blell
Two Women Discovering Urban Cupid,
(triptych), 1979
C prints

Combining the styles of fashion
photography with a conscious
quotation of styles and forms from
art's history, Blell uses the fashion
plate to introduce narrative, romance,
colour and artifice to art photography.

Dianne Blell
Young Woman Overtaken by a Storm,
(triptych), 1979
C prints

Bad hair day. Contravening all the
conventions of 1970s art photography
– naturalness, directness, veracity –
Blell re-stages eighteenth-century
painting, using all the logistical
support, manipulation and
theatricality of the fashion plate.

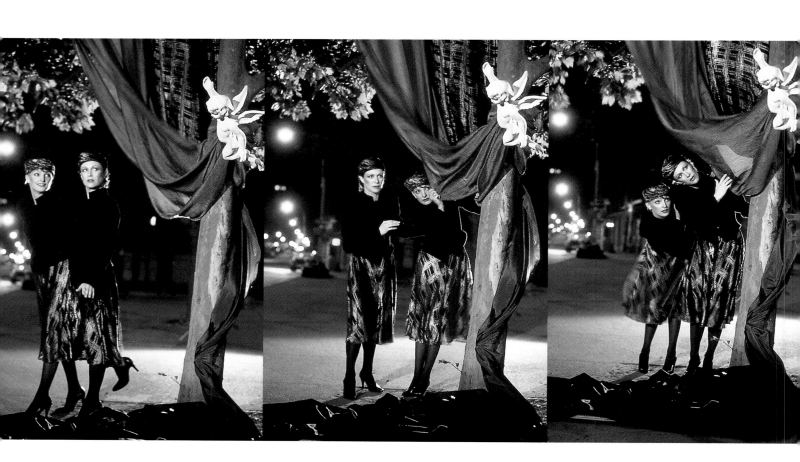

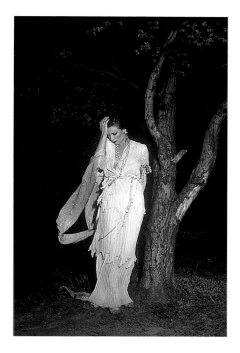
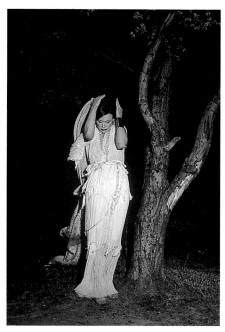
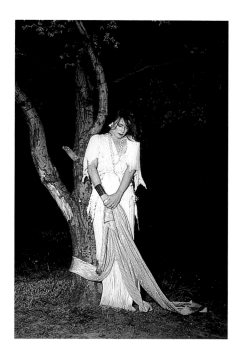

Urban curiosity mingles with apprehension: two young women, richly and strangely attired, peer into the metropolitan terrain at a fleeting, mythological figure. The city enchants. Dianne Blell's triptych of small photographs, *Two Women Discovering Urban Cupid*, 1979, from her series 'Charmed Heads and Urban Cupids', was made in the wake of a cultural upheaval with important consequences for both art and fashion. These images, on the intimate scale and with the palette of Renaissance portraiture rather than the brashness of late twentieth-century colour photography, reflect the impact of this transformation. Where fashion for much of the previous decade had been lost in a wistful rural reverie or else produced a decadent parody of modernity and elegance, its styles and their representation in fashion photography now assumed a harder edge. Responding to the impetus of an aggressive youth culture, fashion became metropolitan, contemporary and, to a degree, less reverently citational. Where art had been critical, and appropriative, in its relationship to fashion and the object in general, it became more citational and incorporative. Following punk's appropriation of art practice, fashion picked up the object of mass culture

and mutilated it; following fashion, art picked up its concerns with formal problems of colour, cut and texture. The ideological agendas of 1970s art softened within practices that acknowledged pleasure, and – like Blell's young urbanites – actively sought it out.

Blell's staged photographs combine the styles of the new fashion photography, manifested especially in the work of Arthur Elgort, with citations from the history of art. In *Two Women Discovering Urban Cupid* the inspiration is Lucas Cranach. Blell remarks that she was especially interested in his symbolically fertile nudes, posed against trees, wearing only an elaborate hat and crowded by swarms of bees.[1] These pictures, and the similarly citational, similarly staged *Young Woman Overtaken by a Storm*, 1979 – where Blell herself assumes a pose from a 1799 painting by Féréol de Bonnemaison – are part of a body of work by young artists that challenges the dominant conventions of art photography. They are in colour; they are staged with models, costumes, make-up artists, hair stylists. All the logistical components of an elaborate fashion shoot are in place rather than the

direct relationship to subject and 'naturalness' insisted upon by the documentary tradition. They compress time: Blell cites the Renaissance and Enlightenment in her images, the Baroque in her gilt frames, and she establishes the photograph as a site for overt recitation when prevailing values insisted only on photography's engagement with the contemporary. These images excavate a history that photography was not meant to possess, recover memories that should belong only to painting. Furthermore, Blell, whilst conceiver of and sometime participant in these scenarios, is neither the exclusive agent of their production, nor 'the photographer'.

Blell's work displays a seductive richness, an investment in the body, its garments and its environments, which is shared with the emerging culture of New Romanticism and learned from late-1970s fashion photography. This is lyrical, tender work, ameliorating the abrasive edge of punk's confrontation with staid values. Blell's work still tells stories of the street, but those narratives are now suffused with sensuality rather than the threat of violence or an insistence on a radically different sexual or racial identity.

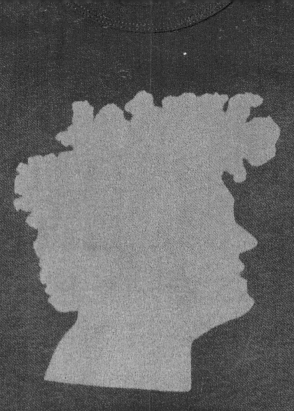

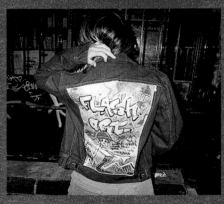

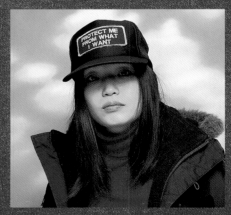

The symbolic (and actual) violence of punk was expressed on clothing through the text and the tear, whether the modified 'I Hate) Pink Floyd' T-shirt, ripped and zipped jeans, or graffitied jacket. Punk style was a conscious iconographic pastiche of older modes of appearance by artfully aware cultural interventionists such as Malcolm McLaren and Vivienne Westwood, and an unstable, continuously modified collection of tropes in which, in lived experience, young punks immersed themselves. As Frank Cartledge, then sixteen and two hundred miles from the King's Road, describes it, 'Locally punk was a crossover between media representations of punk fashion, the commercial clothing available and the 'Do It Yourself", jumble sale, "make and mend" philosophy.'

If the mundane or simply naff could be redeemed for resistance against societal or, at the very least, parental norms through strategies of damage and personalization, so too could art. Rather than an austere supplement to visual assaults on consumerism, 'writing' emerged as a sign of individual presence on the street. As much as for punks scrawling 'Crass' or

'Clash' on leather jackets, this was true for graffiti artists riding New York subway cars and for artists such as Jenny Holzer writing programmatic aphorisms. The venue that mobilized and united the latter two approaches, exhibited them and took them back into culture at street level, was the gallery Fashion Moda, located in the recesses of New York's Bronx. Though not properly part of Manhattan's burgeoning punk scene, many of the young artists nurtured at Fashion Moda would subsequently thrive in that environment, and among the East Village avant-garde it spawned. Stefan Eins founded the gallery in 1972 as a way of taking art into a wider, materially impoverished community. 'Combining the street with the conceptual,'[3] as Eins later described the venture, Fashion Moda recognized graffiti as both a voice of the community and a way of talking to it. Eins provided a platform for the young Keith Haring and Kenny Scharf, as well as locally based artists such as Spank and Lady Pink. Holzer's printed statements – dry confrontations of dominant values – appeared on local lamp-posts and in the gallery window. Soon, however, Eins perceived that the modification of cheap,

ABUSE OF POWER COMES AS NO SURPRISE

Shari Dienes
T-shirt, Documenta, 1982

The culture of the street and the
everyday, transferred, literally,
into an object for high art exhibition.
What starts out as a way of making
art accessible becomes a souvenir
of that radical opening-out for the
art groupie.

Kano
'Flash Art' graffitied jacket, 1984
Lee denim jacket, Krylon and magic
marker on gesso base

A democracy of surfaces and contexts:
the jacket is as suitable a site as a
wall for the graffiti artist's tag. It is
art, worn in the art world, but it is
all about style and nothing to do
with the conventions of the gallery.

Jenny Holzer
'Untitled (Protect Me From What I
Want)' cap, 1982; 'Abuse of Power
Comes As No Surprise' T-shirt,
Documenta, 1982

You've seen the poster; now you can
wear the cap or the T-shirt. Holzer
adapts her artistic strategy to a
moveable, more lasting medium,
and in the process turns conceptual
slogan into art object and fashion
statement.

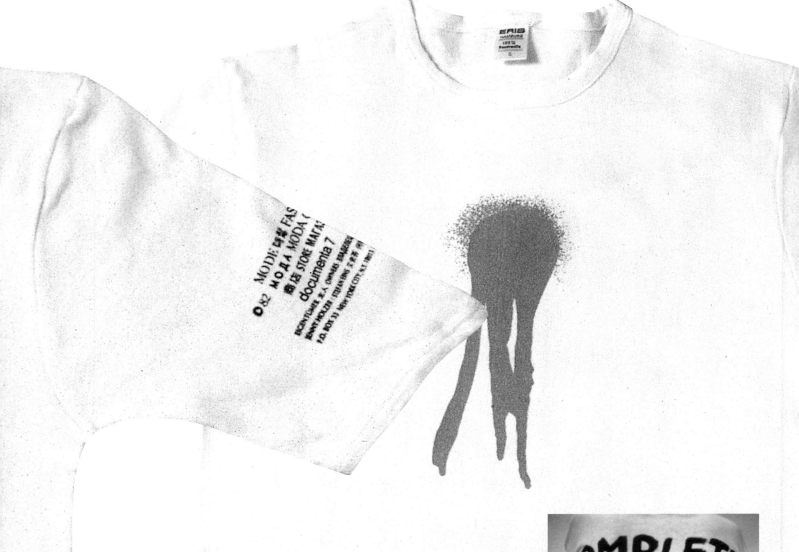

082 MODE FAS...
М О Д А MODA ...
...STORE MAGA...
documenta 7
...HOLZER...
...HOLZER...
P.O. BOX 33 NEW YORK CITY N.Y.1...

46

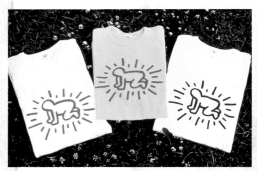

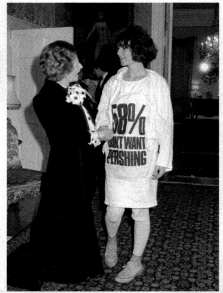

50%
DONT WANT
PERSHING

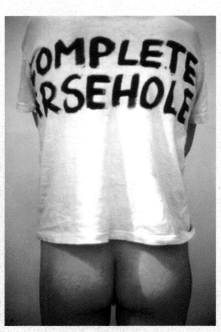

COMPLETE
ARSEHOLE

Stefan Eins
T-shirt, Documenta, 1982

For Eins the T-shirt had been a way
of getting art onto the street in an
impoverished neighbourhood. By
1982 it had found its way into the
art gallery, or at least into the shop.

Keith Haring
T-shirts, Documenta, 1982

Having begun with subway trains and
factory walls, Haring graduated – still
with the same signature figures – to
the increasingly privileged, increasingly
similar surfaces of canvas and catwalk.

Katherine Hamnett
'58% Don't Want Pershing' T-shirt,
(Margaret Thatcher meets Katherine
Hamnett), 17 March 1984

Political statement as fashion, borrowing
an aesthetic strategy from artists such
as Holzer, and returning it to street level.

Tracey Emin and Sarah Lucas
'Complete Arsehole' T-shirt, 1993

The T-shirt as cheap medium for the artist's
edition, and a means of making cheap,
saleable work to sustain young artists.

everyday clothing – a fashion for the streets
and of the streets – represented a significant
medium for these artists.

The graffitied jacket had been an immediate
transformation by, and signification of, its
wearer's unique identity; the modified T-shirt
a statement of individual belief, however
transient. Both art and the fashion industry
quickly saw the potential in formalizing the
strategies of individual sartorial agency.
For Fashion Moda this process reached its
apotheosis at Documenta VII in 1982, when
a group of gallery artists including Holzer,
Haring, Shari Dienes and Eins himself,
produced limited edition T-shirts as
consumable art objects. Other art institutions
quickly pursued the idea: Holzer, for example,
produced both a T-shirt and hat for London's
Institute of Contemporary Arts. At the same
time, however, fashion designers were turning
to 'Holzeresque' expressions of personal
opinion. Katherine Hamnett's collections
of the early 1980s were as much political
slogans as fashion statements, culminating in
her '58% Don't Want Pershing' protest against
British deployment of American nuclear
weapons. The successful young British
designer, a model of business achievement in

a recession-struck country, famously wore this
T-shirt to a meeting with Conservative Prime
Minister Margaret Thatcher, taking fashion into
the place it was least expected to go – politics.
Holzer, at much the same time, was scaling
up her texts, and their 'political' intent,
culminating in a neon billboard display in Times
Square, but for a while both art and fashion
unified in making the billboard for the body.

The model of artist-driven retailing developed
by Fashion Moda, with its roots in Claes
Oldenburg's Pop art project *The Store*, would
persist as an enterprise to which young artists
could resort to sell their ideas, turned into low-
priced editions. The T-shirt as cheap medium
for artwork, made by that art into a statement
of individuality, would likewise remain a staple
of such activities. Amongst the most notorious
of such enterprises was the shop run by Tracey
Emin and Sarah Lucas in East London in the
early 1990s. The self-deprecating irony of their
'Complete Arsehole' T-shirt neatly summarizes
a shift in concerns over a decade of art
practice, from the ideological earnestness of
the early 1980s to a micro-celebrity culture
where individual identity was paramount, even
in its mocking erasure. Fashion, as much as
art, could readily accommodate both extremes.

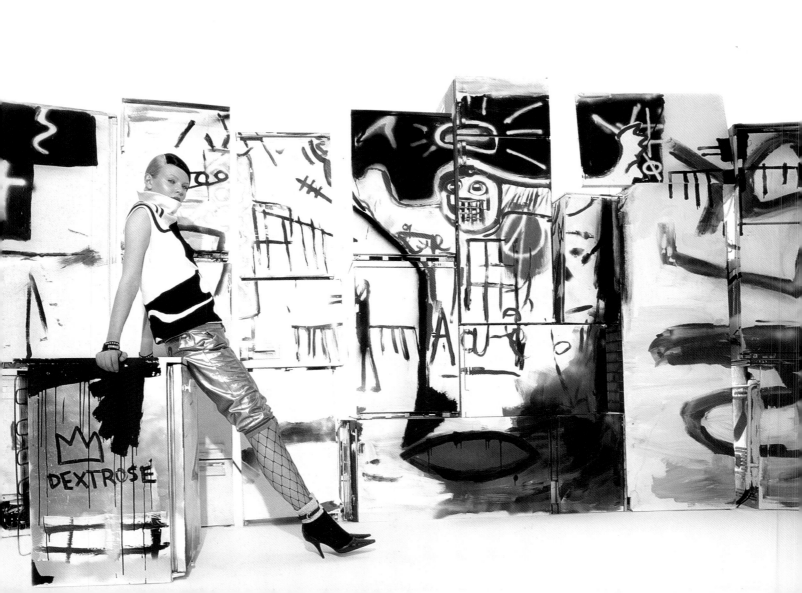

Graffiti – which, regardless of its variable status in the rarefied worlds of art and fashion, remains a fundamental statement of alienated metropolitan identity – became established as a signifier of toughness, of street culture, of 'real' identity. The carefully styled, unauthorized mark became a motif to which fashion designers could repeatedly return as a guarantee of authenticity and individuality through its subversion of the sameness of the manufactured item. This claim on veracity underpins fashion shoots as temporally and thematically distant as Mario Testino's collaboration with Keith Haring for *The Face* in 1984 and Masoud's 'Urban Scrawl' for *Harpers & Queen* at the beginning of 2001. Haring's appearance in one of the leading youth style magazines of the 1980s reflects its editors' abiding interest in the activities of the New York avant-garde, manifested elsewhere in regular reports from the East Village by James Truman. There is, too, a degree of hubris accompanying the invitation to Haring, as the introductory text acclaims a mutual validation between all parties. 'If all stylists are artists and all artists have style, a collaboration between the two on the supremely stylish and artistic fashion pages of *The Face* seemed like a good idea.'[4] Haring's highly stylized trademark figures, which by now were exhibited in upmarket galleries rather than on subway cars, became templates for the re-emergence of the real, as Testino posed models slipping through slits in the painted

Masoud
'Urban Scrawl', *Harpers & Queen*, 2001

The return of the real. The signs of street culture, applied to discarded consumer durables with the same attention to detail manifested in the model's hair and make-up, are appropriated to authenticate high fashion. Art gives bourgeois culture edge. Hasn't this always been the role of the avant-garde?

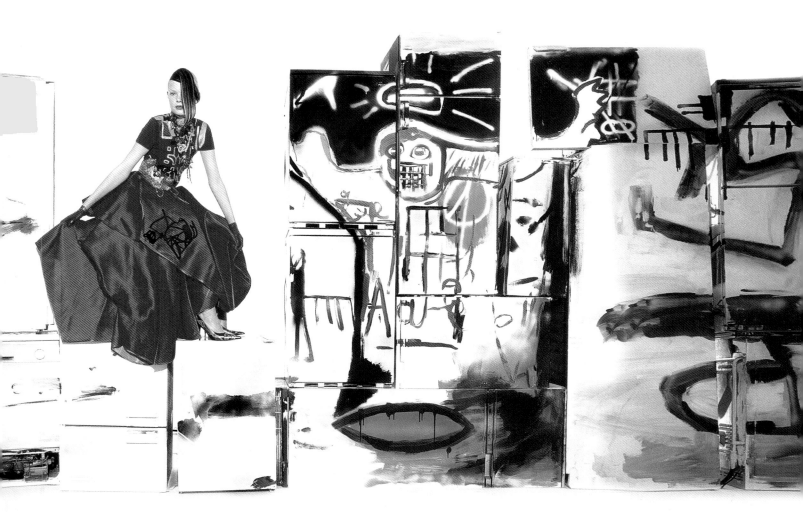

Jean Michel Basquiat
A Panel of Experts, 1984
Mixed media

A self-conscious primitivism
of painting – in which Basquiat
pastiches his own cultural
stereotyping – becomes a
token of street-credibility and
authenticity first for the art world,
and then for fashion mavens.

surface. The drawn, abstracted figure of art functions as a chrysalis from which the authentic figure of street-credible fashion can appear. Neither wholly in nor out, Testino's models occupy a liminal field which mediates between an imaginary world of artistic style and the 'real' environment of fashionable consumption.

Styled by Margherita Gardella, 'Urban Scrawl' not only emphasizes clothing as canvas, in a claim that 'fashion not only reflects art this season, it is art',[5] it also contrasts highly glamorous outfits with graffiti as signifier of urban authenticity. This carefully constructed tautology is a development of Marc Jacobs's gesture of taking a classic Louis Vuitton bag – already a limited-edition, high-quality object – and decorating it with graffiti. Jacobs's defacement, rather than devaluing the object, further enhanced its status through personalization – albeit the designer's rather than the individual owner's. This combination of graffiti and glamour also seems to acknowledge the art world status attained, both in life and posthumously, by artists such as Haring and his fellow casualty of the 1980s, Jean Michel

Basquiat. The discarded fridges and freezers that form the backdrop to Masoud's shoot are decorated in a style that knowingly recalls Basquiat's self-conscious 'primitivism', and one plate even references his citation in its caption.

The *Harpers & Queen* spread exemplifies the circularity of fashion, recalling and modifying 1980s styles: it also subtly suggests the semi-conscious nature of reiteration. In a bitter critique, Theodor Adorno suggested that fashion has no memory. This shoot, however, is not fashion recalling a memory it does not have; rather it suggests a return to attention from the past, accompanied by a consciousness of both the past meanings of the object and the necessity of making the past signify in the changed contexts of the present. Fashion's temporality, rather than being linear, is here shown to be simultaneously circular, following a chain of citations, and progressive, fashioning new meanings from citation. Recalled, the past is not what it was, but rather assumes a new identity which nonetheless acknowledges its history. That art might follow similar trajectories is hinted at by the set's homage to Basquiat.

Artists also go in and out of fashion, and the end of the 1990s and the beginning of a new century have witnessed the reappraisal and rehabilitation of painters such as Basquiat and David Salle, who had shifted from critical valorization to vilification in the previous decade and a half.

If Haring's appearance in *The Face* was a typical manifestation of art's entry into fashion's mediation in the early 1980s, Cindy Sherman's practice in the same period witnessed fashion's entry into art's discourses. Sherman had emerged in the 1970s with images that were simultaneously critical of and, at least in retrospect, rather reverential towards mass-media configurations of femininity. It was no surprise, therefore, that her 1983 exhibition at Metro Pictures should, as Lisa Liebmann put it, 'bring back memories of the photographic layouts that fashion magazines used to run of actresses wearing clothes keyed by the movies that had put them in the big time'.[6] Much of Sherman's early work had referenced and abstracted the look of film stills. A move towards other aspects of cinema's role in purveying an imagination of its identity and encouraging consumption

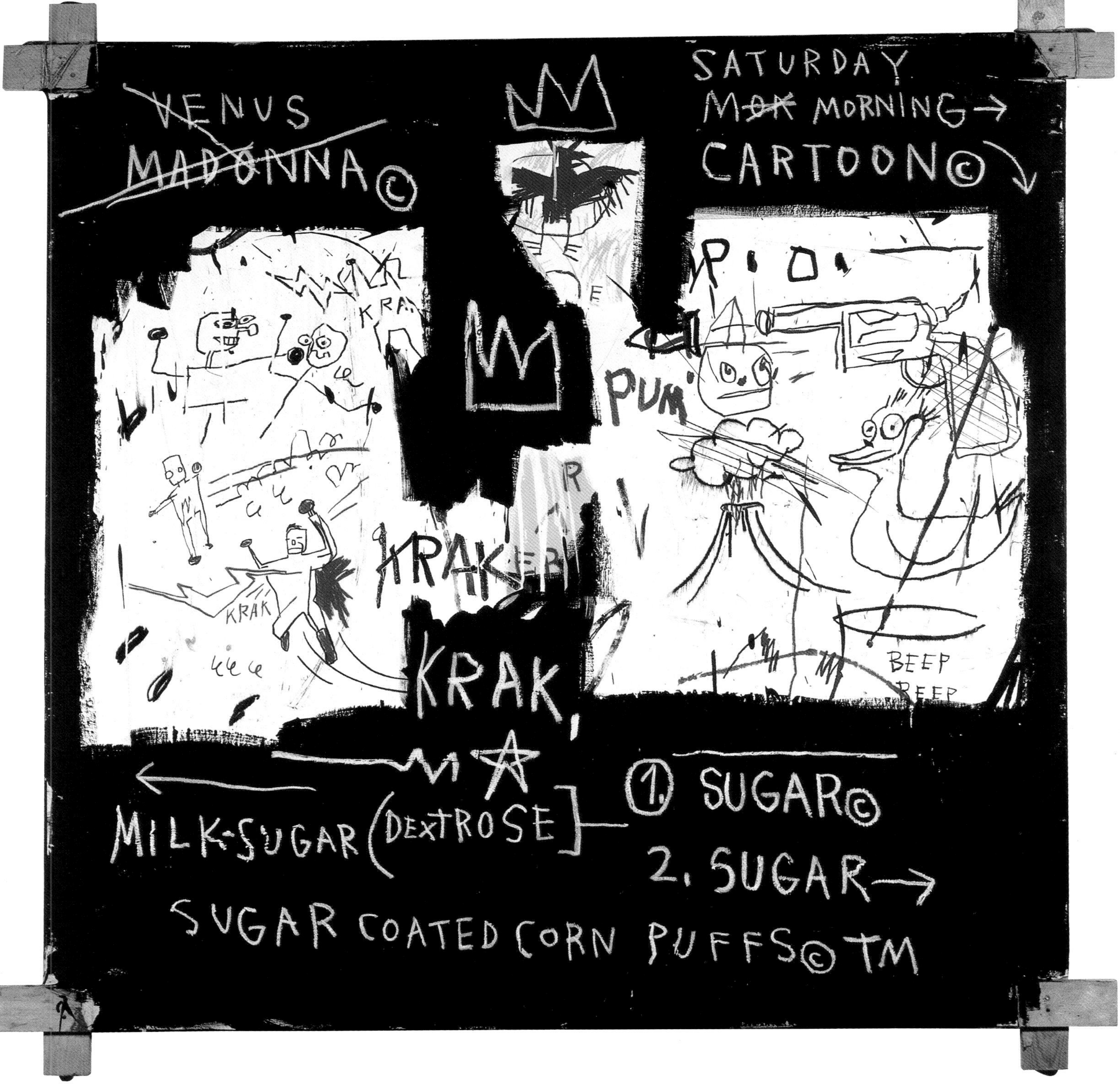
VENUS
MADONNA ©
SATURDAY
MORNING →
CARTOON ©
PUM
KRAK
KRAK
KRAK,
BEEP
1. SUGAR ©
MILK-SUGAR (DEXTROSE)
2. SUGAR →
SUGAR COATED CORN PUFFS © TM

Dressing up, Sherman plays in the boundary zone between art and commerce. Commentaries on the way in which clothing constructs identity are, simultaneously, advertisements for that clothing. At stake is the question of what is meant. Or is it, perhaps, that Sherman has realized the complexity of the relationship? Can art and popular commercial culture be separated? Can art critique and change its 'other', or are the two mutually dependent?

through feminine reimagination and reconfigurations of the self was a logical extension of Sherman's practice.

As Liebmann observed of Sherman's images, this wider focus by the artist signified the growing intimacy of formerly distant cultures. 'Jauntily enough, accurately enough, they consecrate a *renewed* marriage, telling us that fashion has for some time been taking its cues from art, not Hollywood'.[7] Liebmann rightly observed the renewal, rather than the novelty, of the union, but she did not highlight the temporal dynamics of this exchange. Whilst fashion scrutinized, and often took its leads from, contemporary art, art's response had largely been to incorporate fashion into its own histories. The period saw the emergence of the first serious studies of costume history, such as Anne Hollander's profoundly influential *Seeing Through Clothes* and the reappraisal of past fashion photographers including Beaton and Dahl-Wolfe. Accompanying these phenomena was the growth of costume departments in major museums – an interest that arguably stretches well back into modernism's history, with the Metropolitan Museum's 1942 exhibition 'Renaissance in Fashion'.

The alternative approach, for artists such as Sherman, was a critical analysis of the consequences for the individual of that history.

Such a move pulled the historical perspective of Sherman's critique into the sharp focus of the present; her costumed performances within the photograph referenced the emergence of a new generation of designers such as Jean Paul Gaultier, one of whose jump suits was worn by the artist in *Untitled # 131*, 1983. Sherman also directly interpolated her imagery into the discourse of imagination and consumption that she analyzed by producing it in collaboration with a New York fashion retailer, Dianne B, who used a range of the images for advertising purposes. What was, at one level, a critical commentary, became, through the process of its creation, an extension of the subject of its critique. This vertiginous paradox conveyed a sedulously constructed meaning. As Peter Schjeldhal observed, 'We are to know (and she is to know that we know that she knows, in the spiralling complicity of the theatrical) that she is acting an actress acting a part.... We are awash in the force fields of performances not meant for us – this being the sensation meant precisely for us.'[8]

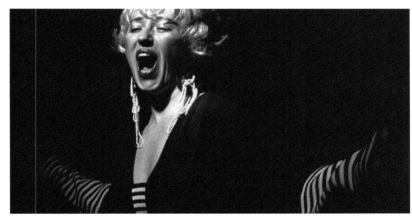

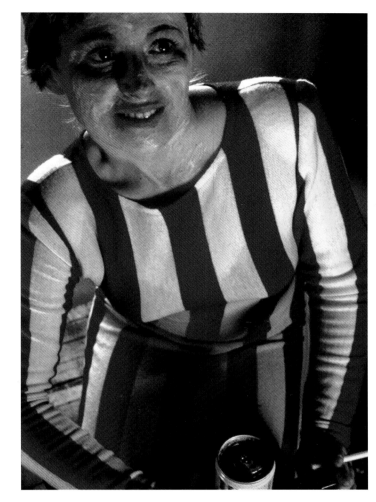

'Model Pleasure', Silvia Kolbowski's series of works from the early 1980s, extracted from, rather than participated in, the performance of the self – or rather, from fashion's solicitations to perform the self. Kolbowski's fractured, fragmentary samples – blissful, pencilled and brushed faces drawn from advertising and fashion shoots – are matched with archetypal metaphors of normative femininity. *Model Pleasure VIII*, 1984, juxtaposes an apple pie – still signifier of feminine domesticity despite its commercial manufacture – with an illustration of an apple variety, 'The Maiden's Blush', with four different pictures of the female face, a panel of text, and a massively enlarged and rotated advertisement from a cheap magazine for a woman's charm anklet. At one level an engaging examination of the social constructions of femininity through visual tropes and textual metaphors, *Model Pleasure* is also a sophisticated analysis of significatory processes.

One of the faces, subject of a beautician's skin peel, is masked under gauze and wraps beside the image of 'The Maiden's Blush', establishing a comparison of exfoliation and consumption whilst reinforcing associations of femininity and fruitfulness. Kolbowski's text cleverly plays with the conjunction of peeling (as a cutting) and desire through a series of erasures and substitutions: 'carved', struck through, becomes 'craved', 'cost' becomes 'cast' – recalling the net of gauze concealing the face in the panel beneath. A close-up of the model's face is striated with white lines which once linked now excised text, object to objective, describing the product and process of shading and highlighting, of colouring and toning, which composed identity. Through these associations Kolbowski suggests that femininity is fashioned from (absent) signs, effectively a construction based upon models of speech, of behaviour, and of their cultural associations, to which we conform. As Craig Owens observed, in a passage that might equally describe the production and cultural deployment of graffiti, these paradigms are effectively cyclical. 'Thanks to the serial disposition of these works ... any image in the series can become the "model" for all the others; conversely, every image in the series is but an imitation of all the others. Thus the "model" is dissolved by the series into a potentially endless repetition of identical gestures and poses. What is at issue, then, is its authority as "model", the supposed inimitability which, paradoxically, makes it imitable.'[9]

Here serial becomes cycle, with the added complication that there is neither guarantee of direction nor order of sequence. Any image may cite or be compared to another, just as fashion, just as art, may reiterate or construct a pose against any moment of its history. Kolbowski's feminist critique of woman's construction also offers not just a model of fashion's, of art's, cyclicality, but of reiteration and cross-reference as cultural condition – integral to signification. Art and fashion both take their lead as cultural products from that more general paradigm of subjectivity, as much as they contribute to its determining effects ●

Silvia Kolbowski
Model Pleasure VIII, 1984
8 photographs (colour and b/w)

'I am all of this, and all of this is me.' Kolbowski's emphasis on complexity and cross-reference illustrates the extent to which culture – and its fashions – construct identity, and the degree to which we think of that culture as nature.

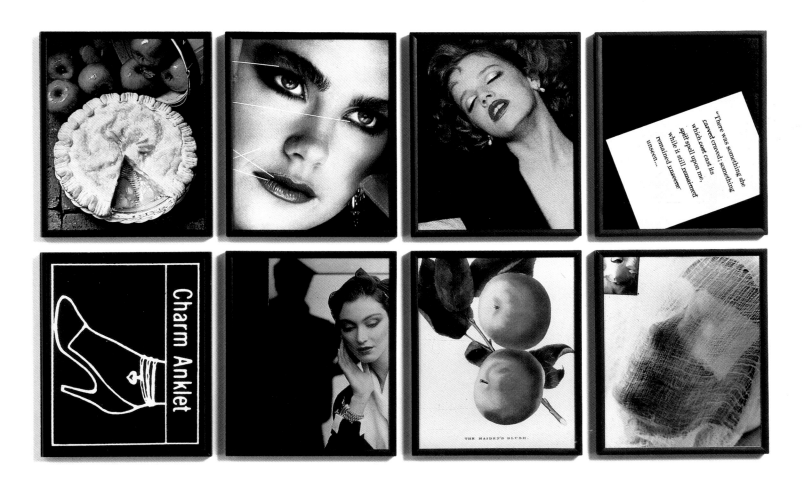

Charm Anklet

"There was something she carved craved; something which cast cast its spit spell upon me, while it still remained remained unseen...

THE MAIDEN'S BLUSH.

3

THE EMPTY BODY
PART 1

IN REPETITION OR
PLAYFUL RETURN,
HOW COULD THE
GHOSTLY CENTRE
NOT CALL TO US?

Jacques Derrida
Writing and Difference

At the beginning of February 1982 the American magazine *Artforum* carried as its cover illustration a photograph of a model wearing an evening dress made by the Japanese designer Issey Miyake. The front cover of *Artforum* had become an increasingly sought-after space within contemporary art; John Coplans, an editor in the 1970s, relates how he was assaulted by an artist desperate for this accolade.[1] The decision to give the cover to Miyake reflected a growing theoretical interest in, and sympathy towards, fashion by the art world. This had been manifested not only in the oeuvres of young artists over the previous five years, but also in expanding critical and historical scholarship and the acquisition of 'canonical' garments by major museums as elements of their curatorial programmes. Whilst much of that scholarly attention had been directed towards the fashion photograph, what appeared on the cover of *Artforum* was not a fashion plate reclaimed from history and popular culture for the purposes of 'high art'. Rather this was an image that highlighted its subject as an object whose formal explorations of colour, shape and texture had fundamental affinities with the interests of contemporary art whilst remaining located in a different register of culture.

Eiichiro Sakata's photograph stressed, through lighting and position, the complex folds and pleats of the fabric, and the exoskeletal architecture of the outfit's rattan bodice. Approached formally, the skirt, with its manifold, torqued layers, seemed like an extension of the ideas of Frank Stella, with his physical complications of representational planes, or the complex tying and pleating of work by Lynda Benglis. That Miyake's surfaces were deeply striated monochromes, edged only by a delicate scarlet piping, seemed to conflate both of Stella's later concerns with the exploration of single colours on shaped surfaces in the artist's early career and the heavily textured, all-black paintings of his great antithesis, Ad Reinhardt. Approached culturally, in relation to the body which the dress both contained and emphasized, its split and contoured carapace suggested a novel positioning of female corporeality: simultaneously erotic, amorous spectacle and armoured, empowered aggressor. A triangle of red beading across the bodice, picking up the line of the wearer's left shoulder, seemed to sew the figure into a structure whose cultural roots were located as much in the technologies of Samurai armour as the more abstracted formalities of Western art.

The foundation stone of an issue of *Artforum* which self-consciously addressed the visible effects of visual art in the public sphere was an editorial by Ingrid Sischy and Germano Celant. Their opening sentences amounted to a frank acknowledgement of the failure of much vanguard art since the late 1960s to achieve its avowed aim of greater accessibility. That ideologically premised intention had too often been accompanied by a withdrawal into hermeticism and an ever more complex and arcane critical infrastructure, in which blindingly simple, and sometimes risible, concepts were presented in language so removed from everyday discourse that only a select few promoted exegetical orthodoxy. This tendency towards 'isolation and conservatism'[2] by an avant-garde which portrayed, and imagined, itself as radical, was understood by Sischy and Celant as a threat to art. In the rigour of its self-scrutiny and the loneliness of its ideological purity, art had largely ceased to be relevant.

To some extent Sischy and Celant were encapsulating the reactions we have already witnessed of young artists to an increasingly academicized conceptualism, but their statement is also prefatory. Presented to historical scrutiny, decades rarely begin or end with clean breaks; far less do such ruptures occur simultaneously in all places in a year ending in zero. (To such an extent is this true, one might argue that periodicity should be reduced to a problematic convention of scholarship and exhibition to be complicated or disavowed even as it is

Issey Miyake
Artforum magazine cover, February 1982

High fashion as high art. On the cover of
the world's most important contemporary
art journal, a Miyake dress is posed
simultaneously as sculpture, as painting
and as aggressive and erotic spectacle;
a signal of transformation in the
relationship of art to mass culture.

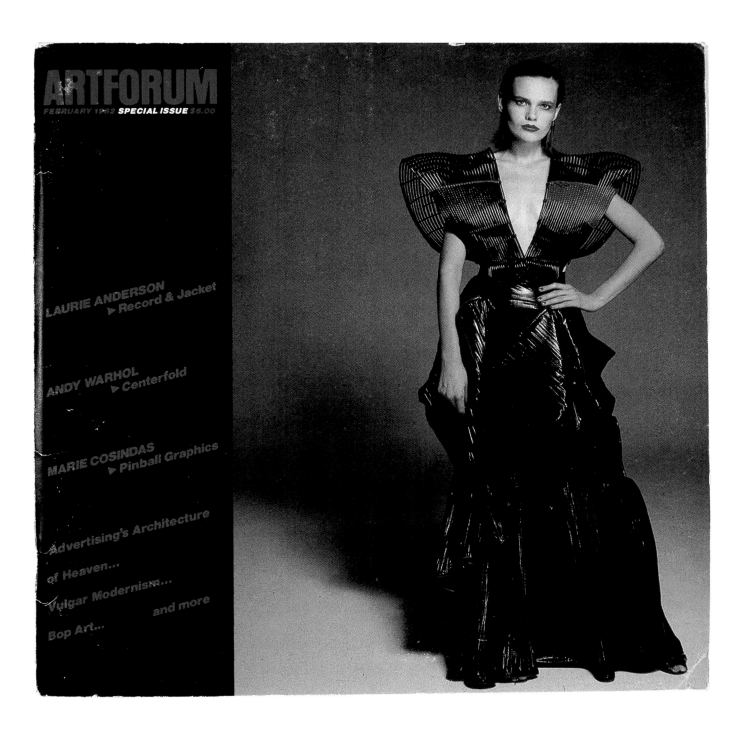

invoked.) The *Artforum* editorial for February
1982 is one sign that ushers in what we
now think of as 'the eighties', with all the
lumber that we retrospectively store in
this abandoned room of our experience.
In particular the co-authored text signals
important changes in the concerns of art
and its relationship to mass culture.

Sischy and Celant presciently suggested
that art was one element in a far larger
system of visual culture and communication
– which their decision to feature Miyake's
designs immediately acknowledged as
including fashion – and that there was 'a
changing dynamic between the language
of the avant-garde and the vulgate, both of
which seem to be feeding on each other'.[3]
A decade earlier *Artforum* had established
much of its pre-eminence on a willingness
to recognize connections between different
visual domains. The journal had, however,
become affected by the same introspection
that permeated art in the 1970s, even as
it diversified the media of its practice and
proclaimed itself open and accessible.
Sischy and Celant called for a renewal of
that contract, with a recognition that the
dynamic existed, and an understanding
that to be a dynamic it *must* change. This
reiteration of art and culture's engagement
was to be facilitated through a renewed
relationship to the object, whether that was
the commodity of mass culture, embraced

by Pop art, or the body, no longer
understood as monumental index but
as manipulable, plastic sign of personal
narrative. Sischy and Celant point to an art
that is, quite literally at times, impure and
haptic. Many artists in the 1980s responded
to art's piety by participating in an unclean,
noisy world. Unlike, say, Philip Guston in
the early 1970s, returning directly to
the subjects of history through the mass-
cultural medium of the cartoon, many of
them got their hands dirty by delving into
the worlds of commerce and mass
signification.

Sischy and Celant suggested a shared
circularity within art and fashion dependent
on the 'manipulation of preceding "models"'
and 'continual, reckless ingestion of the
phantom of history'.[4] This commitment to
the perpetually modern necessitates not
only the rejection of the past – for fashion,
long after the era of high modernism,
remains relentlessly committed to the
dictum to 'make it new' – but also, through
the occlusion of history, the guarantee of
its return. As Herbert Blau puts it, 'At the
same time that fashion would seem to be
the datum of postmodernity, or its generic
domain, it also perpetuates the cultural
logic of late modernism, whose most
radically sustained investment is the
tradition of the new.'[5] The choice of Miyake's
1982 collection as a point of incision into art
and mass culture's circularity is of symbolic
value, but in making that point the editors
necessarily overlook prior engagements
within art that, appropriating fashion,
already employed a concern with form to
critique the cultural location of the body.

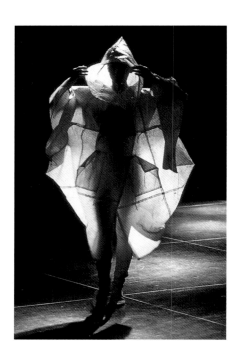

Lynda Benglis
Untitled, 1982
Wire, plaster, gold leaf

Gilding and twisting, Benglis uses
sculptural form as an analogy for
both fabric and the dynamics of the
body that might shape and bear it.
The under-structure becomes the
substance of the absent object.

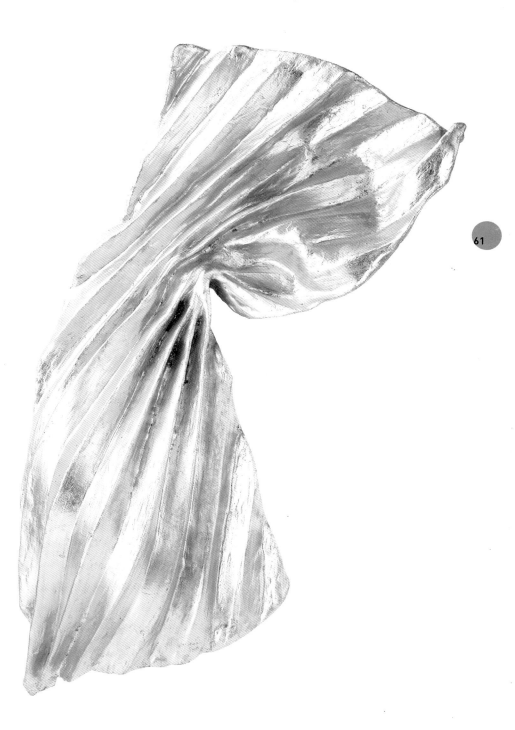

Maureen Connor's series of sculptural
works made in 1981, including *Inside Out*,
Undertitled and *Birth of the Bustle* were
constructed with much the same materials
as Miyake used in his 1982 collection:
reeds, paper and silk. Connor's project
had no temporal precedence over Miyake's.
As Laurence Bénaïm observes, Miyake's
practice from 1968 to 1998 depended upon
a use of 'the often abstract volume of the
garment to hide or mask the body, for the
sake of making a distinction between
them'.[6] An interest in heterological
conjunction – the sustaining of distinction
rather than dialectical resolution – is
emphasized in Miyake's designs by the
presence of a body as armature. In Connor's
oeuvre a similar heterology is realized
through absence: the carapace becomes an
evocative trace of the elided body. Similarly,
the work of Lynda Benglis – one of the few
artists to retain an interest in colour and
form through the 1970s – reflected new
preoccupations with the body at the end of
that decade. These appear first in pieces
such as *Megiste*, 1978, where Benglis gilds
voluptuous and distended torsos, but from
1979 the sense of embodiment conveyed by
the corporeal is displaced into an attention
paid to folded, twisted, skeletal under-
structures. As Susan Krane notes of
sculptures such as *Fanfarinade*, 1979,
and *Mirtak*, 1983, 'In spite of their
anthropomorphic and often anatomical

61

references, these objects lack all bodily presence, as if they were pure fanciful artifice or apparition.[7]

Sischy and Celant's text examines critically the thesis put forward by certain of modernism's proponents of a dialectic between autonomous art and mass culture. 'A reciprocal hierarchical order was established based on this opposition between serious and frivolous, high and low, pure and impure. These distinctions were determined by a dialectic between esthetic and utilitarian values, between the unique and the multiple, between the useless and useful, between elite and vulgar.'[8] The *Artforum* editors point to Pop art as fundamentally deconstructive of such distinctions. However, we might see in Miyake's, Connor's and Benglis's shared insistence on the sustained and mutually antagonistic presence of irreconcilable oppositions a similar dismissal of dialecticism, without recourse to a reconfiguration or relocation of the mass-cultural object.

Roland Barthes remarked that 'the incapacity to name is a good symptom of disturbance'.[9] Connor's *Undertitled* is almost that symptom – a work which in its proper deconstruction of not-naming (proper in that it dismantles and differently reassembles) deploys a title that undertakes the same project as the object which it does name. Early reviews of Connor's pieces understood them as clothes that could not be worn: after all, they looked like the bleached, skeletal remains of Victorian corsets. In some senses that conclusion was correct: to attain use value these sculptures demanded an impossible body. This, in part, was Connor's intention: a commentary on the social imposition of the morphology of bodies. The sculpture's deconstruction of

the object removed the figure from apprehension. However, the enigmatic spectacle of reconfiguration simultaneously drew attention to that absence – after all, there *should* have been a body there. This gesture reintroduced what was missing as the subject of attention.

Undertitled, and its companion piece *Inside Out*, highlight one of Connor's principal strategies in effecting a corrosion of dialectical terms. What were once under and inside are now over and out. There is an inversion of parietal surfaces. As with Miyake's deliberate exposure and armouring of the torso, there is here a displacement of the skeletal structure. Fashion and art's mutual disturbance of hierarchical privilege, making the armature of the body into a spectacle unsupported by any (visible) architecture, and especially Connor's emphasis upon an equivalence of surface, enacts that disordering of spatial ontology theorized by Jacques Derrida in his essay *Fors*.[10] Here, subjective interiority – the hidden structural condition of being –

is called to the surface and made obvious as a particular effect upon and within both body and soul, which is otherwise effaced by our attention to surface appearances. Combining the Latin *foris* (outside) with the French *for intérieur* (inner heart), the idea of the *fors* permits an imagination of surface where the two, seemingly opposing terms, are constitutive of each other. Connor's works may demand an impossibly convulsed body, but the condition of the corset makes it clear that this exaggerated corporeality is only a little more extreme than the material limits to which the female body has already been pushed and pulled by peculiar discursive pressures. The writing *on* the body that is fashion's imposition is revealed as a hidden writing *of* the body, a conformance to corporeality to which we subscribe.

An extension of this preoccupation with interiority and its revelation is central to Zizi Raymond's work of the late 1980s and early '90s. Having experimented with found objects, Raymond sought 'a more figurative presence in the work'.[11] This presence, as for Connor and Benglis, was achieved through the paradox of absence. Shoes and clothes became substitutes for their possible wearers. Raymond's concern is with the social and historical role of clothing, its coding of the subject as a kind of uniform; a means of identification which also camouflages difference and dissent; a signifier of limited, predictable behaviour. Raymond resituates obvious, universal

below
Maureen Connor
Inside Out, 1981
Reed, silk ribbon

below right
Maureen Connor
Undertitled, 1981
Reed

Connor's early works are structures that demand an impossible body. They reconfigure the skeletal imposition of the corset as if it was the body itself – transforming what should be a concealed armature into spectacle.

below
Issey Miyake
Wire body, autumn/winter 1983/84

What was once a vessel of containment becomes a surface of partial revelation and display. Miyake's constructions do not hold in the body; they extend its surface, reinforce its allures.

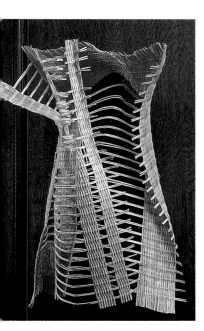

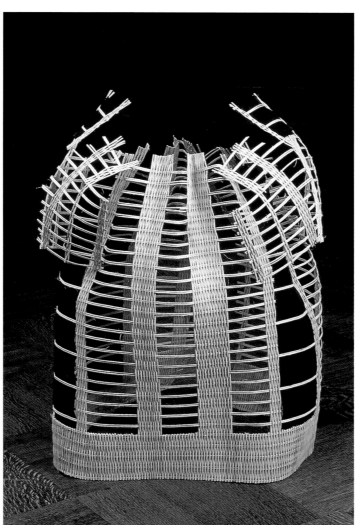

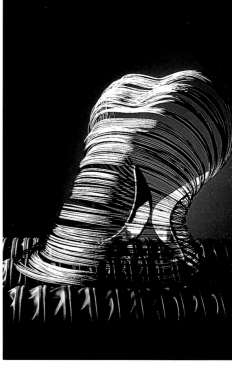

Zizi Raymond
Untitled (Undertow), 1989
Bathing suit, thread, stones

A visual paradox: Raymond creates both
a swimsuit that would sink a body and one
that would blend it into the beach. It is not
so much a swimsuit as camouflage.

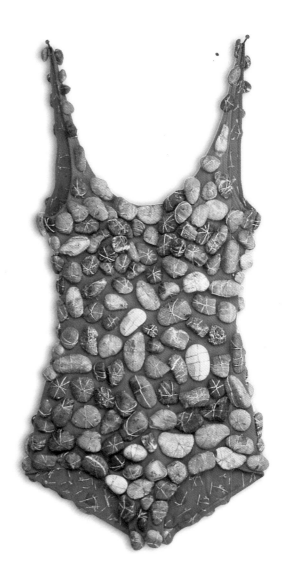

items of clothing in a hinterland where they
are poised between presence and absence,
and also, as the artist observes, 'between
humour and menace'.[12] Like Connor's pieces
of the early 1980s, Raymond's work
with fashion undermines the dialectical
propositions of modernism, which would
maintain fashion's frivolous, subordinate
status. Rather than bringing the subordinated
term to attention, however, Raymond shifts the
obvious, the historically privileged, to a space
where it teeters continually on the brink of
disappearance and appearance, as in *Hiding*,
1990, or, as in the stone-covered swimsuit
of *Undertow*, 1989, where it demarcates a
boundary between utility value and
uselessness.

Connor's *Birth of the Bustle*, in its title, points
towards an underlying structure, a residue
that might form the semi-prosthesis of a
weighted, grotesquely extended dress.
Once again the skeletal becomes pellicular.
This naming, in its reference to a long-
obsolete clothing style, designed to modify
and hamper the movement of the body,
now seems strangely anticipatory. The bustle,
having gone the way of the corset, would soon
make a reappearance in the knowing catwalk
citations of Vivienne Westwood, renegotiated
as simultaneously a commentary on its status
as object of female repression and as an
emphatic statement of scale. In a bustle you
can't escape presence. Benglis, at much the
same time as Connor, was thinking of her
work *Cassiopeia*, 1982, as 'a bustle'.[13] *Birth of
the Bustle* is a sign of *re*birth; a suggestion not
only of continual recitation – that omnivorous
appetite of fashion for its own past – but also
that the structural imperatives which created
the original bustle remain unchanged, even if
clothed in different forms, or perhaps not
clothed at all.

Zizi Raymond
Hiding, 1990
Paper, twine, shoes

Blanking the body. What is meant to be revealed through clothing disappears behind raw fabric. Clothing becomes an inadequate substitute for a regressing human subject.

Maureen Connor
Birth of the Bustle, 1981
Reed, organdy paper

What had been an underlying structure to extend the body is reborn as freestanding, sculptural form with its own skin and its own identity. Inside becomes outside, but also the obsolete becomes novelty.

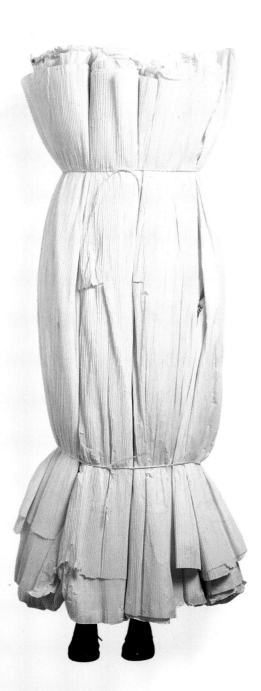

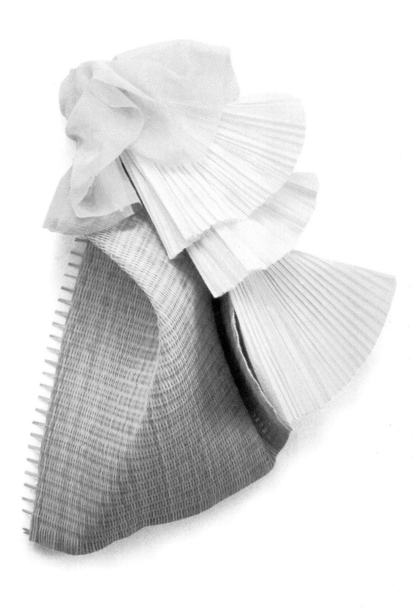

Jean Paul Gaultier
Classique fragrance bottles,
launched 1993

The symbol of bodily repression and
constraint becomes the signature of
creative rebellion. Gaultier makes
the corset into a sign of eroticism and
unique identity for the consumer – and
sells it inside an ordinary tin can.

**Madonna in Jean Paul Gaultier
corset, 'Blonde Ambition' tour, 1990**

The constraining, private object becomes
public spectacle. There is nothing
about the Gaultier corset that is holding
Madonna in place. In a parallel with
the reversals instigated by Maureen
Connor, it is the body that sustains
the exterior.

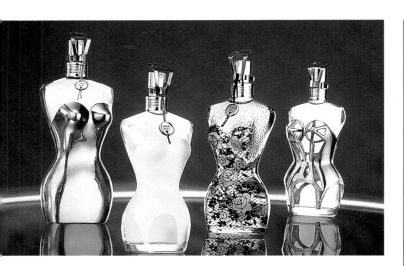

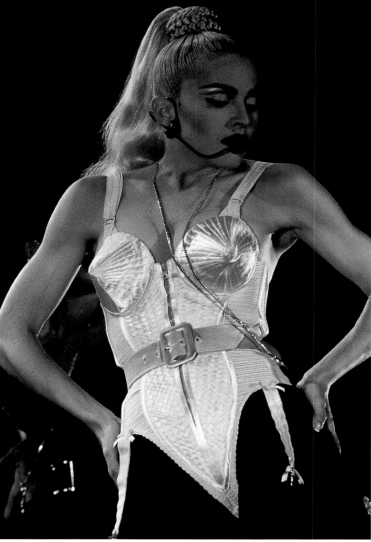

66

Vivienne Westwood
'Nymphs' leather strapless dress,
spring/summer 2002

The corset – strapless in Westwood's
designs – channels and sexualizes
the body. It returns to its old role, but
Westwood ensures that part of the erotic
charge derives from its flagrant display.

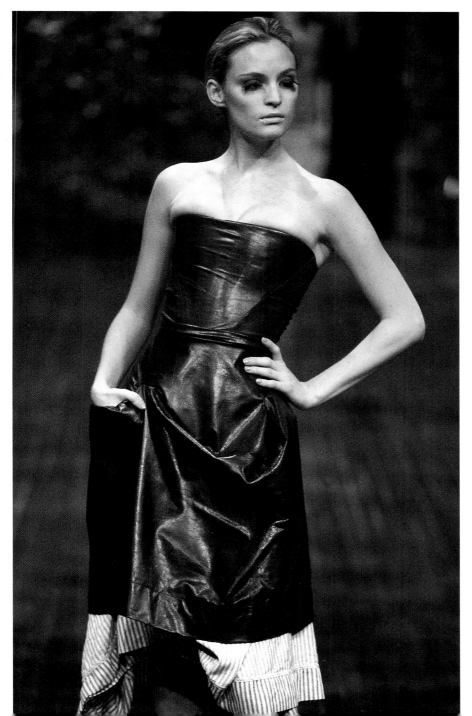

The reinventions of fashion would lead
Westwood and Jean Paul Gaultier to recognize
that the constraints of corsetry and the bustle
also possessed a certain flagrant, liberating,
erotic effect. Binding and hobbling drew
attention to the body as spectacle, a body that
artists could not bring themselves to present,
but which fashion demanded. In these
historical re-presentations both Gaultier and
Westwood would self-consciously cite art
history as an integral component, Gaultier
choosing Dada, and Westwood in the early
1990s invoking the sexual and economic excess
and imaginary bucolic dalliances of pre-
revolutionary France through her use of
Boucher. Designers and artists, through the
clothing of restraint, seemed to imagine a
common, hyperbolic body which might wear
such garb. Artists perhaps contemplating this
figure with horror rendered it impossible
and/or absent; designers dared to imagine the
monstrous 'engineering' which might make it
practicable. The 1980s were, of course, a
decade that would continually produce
'spectacular' bodies, whether in the inflated
torsos of Schwarzenegger, Stallone and the
'muscle Mary', the over-emphatic corporeality
of the supermodel, or, antithetically, the
debilitated musculature of those with AIDS.

Gaultier would symbolize the transformative
possibilities of inscribing (or at least binding
and wiring) the body – its movement from the
quotidian to the spectacular – in a mass object
rather than a fashion item. A bottle of eau-de-
toilette, its flesh-pink glass blown and frosted
in the shape of a corseted torso, emerged from
an ordinary tin can. Clad in Gaultier and finely
attuned as ever to the cultural pulse, in 1990 –

only ten years after the emergence of the body as subject – Madonna, with her 'Blonde Ambition' tour, would recapitulate what was already, or had been, spectacle as spectacle. A so-very-eighties somatic fashioning would highlight the salient points of the discourse for those whose attention had somehow been elsewhere for the previous decade. Just as Sischy and Celant acknowledged the movement of artists towards the objects of mass culture after the fact, so mass culture, in the form of Madonna, retrospectively registered the body as object. In hypothesizing a fine art practice which commingled with the vernacular, the *Artforum* editors perhaps over-emphasized what was already mass-cultural as a reaction to the elitism of 1970s art. They also overlooked a convergence of interests, on both sides of the divide they sought to dismantle, that already addressed the body as visible commodity. Sischy and Celant never acknowledged that mass culture could fail as easily as art, even if it failed differently. The metamorphoses

of discourse around the body throughout the '80s would demonstrate that, just as readily as the genres of elitist art, globally accessible mass-media forms, including the music spectacular, could spectacularly – and as spectacle – miss the point.

More perspicacious was Valerie Steele's insight that 'the corset did not so much disappear as become transformed, first into girdles, bustiers and brassières; and then – more radically – it became internalised through diet and exercise. The hard body replaced the boned body.'[14] Wearing a Gaultier corset, Madonna condensed a half-decade's conversion of puppy-fat into muscle in a metonymical figure which also represented a convulsion of surface – musculature worn on the outside, as it were. This literalization of the unseen had, effectively, been Connor's strategy a decade before – except that Connor's structures also referred beyond themselves to a constricting ideological construct of the female body which the corset, in its historic configurations, helped enforce. The absent bodies to which Connor's work, with that of Benglis and latterly Raymond, referred had not, however, disappeared into the ether. As Steele suggests, they rematerialized as container rather than contained. This new register of the body – mould rather than contents – is underscored in Julie Major's

torsos of the mid-1990s, which equate weight and volume with the body, not burying the structure of the subject but cohering it as mass. In *Untitled (after Gabrielle d'Estrées and her sister)*, 1996, Major would gesture towards a specific femininity and naturalness for these 'bodies', but at all times her use of 'fashioning' devices as analogues for the body emphasizes the solidity and rigidity of the corpus which fills and contours fashion, rather than the exoskeleton which once conformed it ●

Julie Major
Untitled (after Gabrielle d'Estrées and her sister), 1996
Flock, leather, coldcast aluminium

The garment opens to reveal itself as ripening body. Major coheres the corset and its contents as a single fecund mass. In her hands sculpture is at once ethereal and corporeal; both promise and discovery.

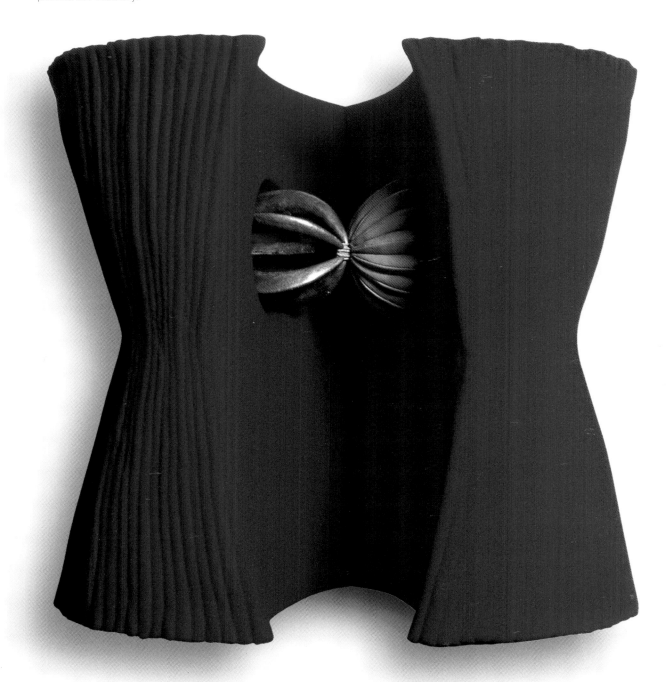

4

THE EMPTY BODY
PART 2

SKIN HAS NO EDGES.
CLOTHES DO.

Peter Schjeldhal
Village Voice, April 1991

Judith Shea's large studio occupies part of an industrial building in Queens. Sandwiched between electrical distributors and clothing wholesalers, it offers a spectacular view of mid-town Manhattan. The studio is only a few blocks from PS1, the gallery where, in 1976, Shea installed work in a group show that was to have considerable significance for both participating artists and institution. PS1 had been a New York school. Shut down in 1964, a decade later it began to be used as a space for new art. Refitting for this purpose was, however, minimal; indeed, non-existent. One review of PS1's opening described it as 'the apotheosis of the crummy space'.[1] Both gallery and contents deliberately represented a zero degree of statement about art and its institutions. If it was an apotheosis, then it was an inversion, a low point as mark of success. For the post-minimalist generation, space and art were so self-effacing, so self-erasing, that they were simultaneously invisible and profoundly revealing about the processes and gestures of making a mark, about the presence of art in time and (crummy) space.

Shea had been trained in fashion design, and spent the early 1970s producing one-offs for leading department stores such as Henri Bendel. Her extemporizing methods seemed to anticipate the punk aesthetic that would emerge only a few years later, but we might discern in both this improvisation and the already sculptural properties it embodied, a concern with dimension and temporality that recurs in the work of Elisa Jimenez in the late '90s. These interests also anticipate the formal shifts of Shea's own career as an artist which exemplify a re-embodiment of art through fashion and a recourse to narrative in its forms. A few years later Richard Flood would observe, 'That Shea's garments from the mid-seventies remain so impervious to time, so symbiotically linked to her current sculpture is both satisfying in itself and in that it defies traditional notions of genre. Her art is derived from a software vocabulary that has everything to do with fashion, and is only marginally related to the common art-historical references. Shea's major point of personal reference is rooted in the anthropology of clothing construction.'[2]

'Rooms' at PS1 represented a shift of those concerns away from the structured spaces of retail fashion to the deconstructed architecture of an art gallery made as distant from the aesthetics and politics of the white cube as it was possible to get and still be reviewed in *Artforum*. Much of what went on in PS1 directly concerned itself with the improvised rearticulation of primary materials, whether the structure of the gallery itself in Richard Nonas's rusted steel beam stretched down a corridor and Gordon Matta-Clark's untitled cut into the floors; the dimensional vectors of art's making (time and space) in Michelle Stuart's *East/West Wall Memory Relocated*; or the fundamental materials of art's making, which were Shea's choice. Shea did not paint her canvases. She left the heavy material raw and shaped it into garments which took their reference from construction – cutting, stitching and folding where more traditional sculptural materials might be welded or moulded – and using the discrepancy between architecture and inhabitant to emphasize a separation between body and object. This resort to fashion as a primary structure offered a commentary on the relationship of nature and culture unusual in post-minimalism, and rarer still within fashion, though Martin Margiela's generic size 74 collection of 2000 has evinced similar interests. Shea accentuated this concern by a displacement of the objects into a register of use value – what Flood divined as her interest in the anthropological. *King and Queen*, 1976, became something other than 'art' when it was taken down from the wall and worn at the exhibition's opening party by the diminutive Dorothy and Herbert Vogel (see p. 17).

If Shea's PS1 exhibit represented a refashioning of art's most primary materials in fashion's most elemental structures, her next project took that 'minor' element of the artist's oeuvre – the work on paper – and made it into a work *of* paper. *New Urban Landscape # 9*, 1977, a 'project to affect the urban landscape of Lower Manhattan' was commissioned by the Institute for Art and Urban Resources, a Manhattan-based organization which, in addition to raising much of the capital for PS1, funded artworks within the public domain rather than the more sanctified spaces of the gallery and museum. Shea presented the Institute with a folded, printed sheet of paper. The text briefly described who Shea was, what the Institute did, and how to make the sheet of paper into a wearable garment. A photograph printed on one side showed an idealized version of how instruction – process – realized itself as art.

Mark Borthwick
Chloë Sevigny modelling pieces from Martin Margiela's size 74 collection, spring/summer 2000

A perfect fit. Emphasizing the separation between body and object – a gap which most fashion seeks to close – Martin Margiela creates a range that everyone, and no one, can wear.

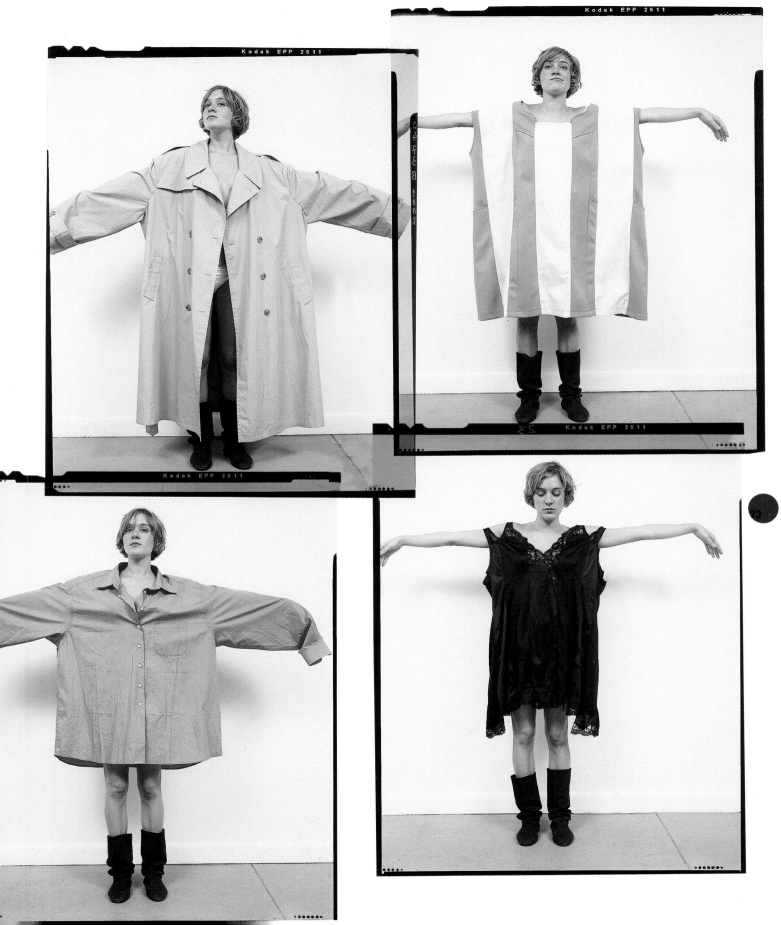

The sheet was distributed within the districts of Lower Manhattan. This strikingly simple work made sculpture and fashion out of primary art material, but it also emphasized the fragility and ephemerality of the latter by challenging the traditional durability and solidity of the former.

From this point of reductivity, Shea would use fashion to reconfigure her personal artistic language. The canvas jacket pieces made in the wake of the PS1 exhibition and *New Urban Landscape # 9*, were at first similarly concerned with flatness and shape. These geometrical forms began to introduce colour – or, rather, monochrome. One piece in the series used black ink, silkscreened over the canvas, another grey pastel applied laboriously by hand. Colour followed shortly after, in a series whose geometrical shapes derived from the simplified outlines of shirts, dresses, coats and sleeveless tops. Unlike the canvas jackets, however, these works had lost their limited anthropological value: they were no longer wearable, though they seemed still to refer to some distant, abstracted corporeality. Hung from dowels and stained or dyed with primary colours, pieces such as *"Judy"*, *"Peggy"*, *"Kathy"*, 1980, were effectively monochromes which, had they been realized in paint on more artistically privileged surfaces than taffeta or silk organza, might have been linked to the formal exercises in colour and shape undertaken by Ellsworth Kelly. Instead, Shea's new work, coupled in a review with Maureen Connor's first solo exhibition, was most publicly discussed in terms of craft and seen only as an exploration of clothes that could not be worn.[3] More perceptive commentaries placed Shea both in a tradition of 'sabotaged utilitarianism', exemplified in recent women's art by Pat Lasch and Cynthia Carlsson, and an internal critique of post-minimalism,[4] whilst Ronny Cohen recognized that Shea, uniquely, was 'dealing with fashion as structure and form rather than decoration and image'.[5]

Whilst Matisse was an obvious point of reference for these cut and coloured shapes, the interest in structure that Cohen discerned signalled other, more radical precursors. There is something of the Russian Constructivist aesthetic about the primary colours and dynamic shapes. Their diffused use value still points to a social relevance, and it is perhaps no coincidence that at this time

opposite
Judith Shea
New Urban Landscape # 9, 1976
(view of the artist wearing the edition as a shirt)
Paper

The fundamental substrate of drawing and painting – the sheet of paper – is made into both sculpture (through the introduction of dimension) and a parody of everyday, briefly wearable fashion.

below
Judith Shea
Studio view, 1979–80

Flattened against the studio wall, fashion is reduced to shape, colour and texture. Dimension will come later. For now Shea's recourse to fashion's formal elements both challenges and extends the post-minimalist obsession with art's rhetorical forms.

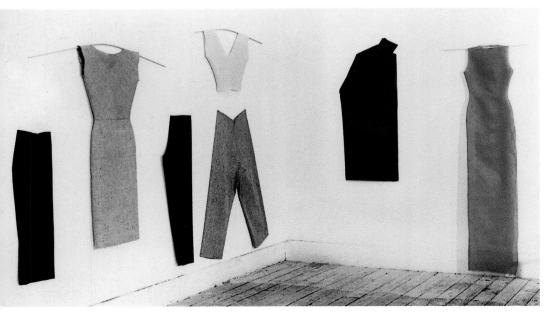

INSTITUTE FOR ART AND URBAN RESOURCES
Executive offices: 108 Leonard Street,
New York City 10013

Projects:
THE CLOCKTOWER, 108 Leonard St., N.Y.C.
CLOCKTOWER, center of the Institute
P.S.1 (PROJECT STUDIOS ONE), 21-01 46th Rd., L.I.C.
Long Island City center for the Experimental
Arts.
...space program at The Clocktower, P.S.1,
and 10 Bleecker Street.

...grateful to the 'Friends of the Institute', John Comfort, Chairman, for making possible
...and other publications from the series.

...artists representing a wide variety of disciplines
...Lower Manhattan to the people who live and work there.
...with partial funding from the City Spirits Program of the National
...en), with the cooperation and supervision of the Office of Lower Manhattan
...en, Director, and the New York City Department of Cultural Affairs.

Project to affect the urban landscape of lower Manhattan.
Tear collar 3 5/8" x 13" off this edition.
Slash down center 8 3/4".
Fold up pocket.
Tape, glue, staple, tab and slot or otherwise join all pieces (see photo).
Wear.

January, 1977

INSTITUTE FOR ART AND URBAN RESOURCES, 108 Leonard Street, New York City 10013; (212) 233-1096

President: Alanna Heiss • Vice-President: Linda Blumberg

EXECUTIVE STAFF

BOARD OF DIRECTORS
Brendan Gill, Chairman • Lawrence Alloway • John Hightower • Jerald Ordover • Robert Rauschenberg.

FRIENDS OF THE INSTITUTE
John Comfort, Chairman • Mr. & Mrs. Oliver W. Bivons • Mr. & Mrs. Pieter Van de Bovenkamp • Melissa
Cooper, Brandt • Mr. & Mrs. Leo Castelli • Ms. Mary Lea D'Arc • Donald Droll • Virginia Dawn •
James I. Elliot • Mr. & Mrs. Ronald Feldman • Mr. & Mrs. Paul Frankel • Mr. & Mrs. Albert Hirschmann •
Klaus Kertiss • Christophe de Menil • Mr. & Mrs. Mony Money Robert Moyal • Mr. & Mrs. David Robinson •
Robert Stefanotty • Harry Torczyner • Ms. Berta Walker • Mr. C. David Robinson •
Mr. Daniel Silberberg • Mr. & Mrs. Andrew Fuller.

NEW URBAN LANDSCAPES
a focus on lower manhatt[an]
of documented projects.

opposite
Judith Shea
Black Dress, 1983
India ink on wool felt, wood plinth

Recognizably a figurative sculpture, Shea's work nonetheless challenges the conventions of the mode through its choice of materials and the absence of a body. Its trace emphasizes the ephemerality of that which the monument makes permanent.

right
Judith Shea
"Judy", "Peggy", "Kathy", 1980
Silk organza

Shea undertakes formal exercises in monochrome colour and shape that owe a stylistic debt to Matisse and the Russian Constructivists.

below
Judith Shea
Black Jacket, 1979
Silk-screened ink on canvas organza

Responding perhaps to Ad Reinhardt or Frank Stella's early work, Shea's take on the monochrome moves from spirituality to corporeality, from non-meaning to subjective meaning. She achieves this not on canvas as fixed surface, but through canvas as potential costume.

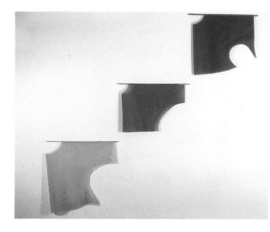

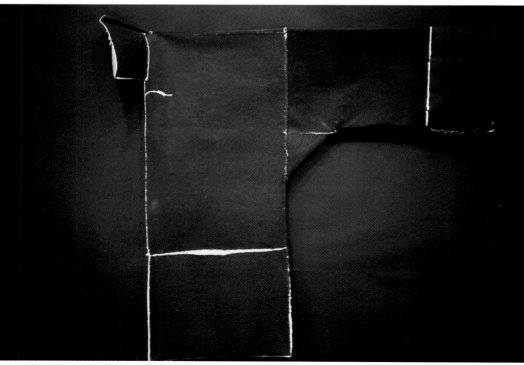

Shea was also making costumes for Trisha Brown's dance company and performances staged by the poet Ted Greenwald. Constructivist artists of the Communist revolutionary era had similarly combined their formal explorations of artistic language in shape and colour with theatrical costuming. Shea in the early 1980s shared affinities with a group of modernist artists which included not only women avant-gardists such as Alexandra Exter, Liubov Popova and Varvara Stepanova, but also male contemporaries including Kazimir Malevich, who were attempting to synthesize formal experimentation with a utopian political vision. Shea was not pursuing such an overtly radical agenda with her work. The revivification of Constructivist aesthetics here allowed the artist to escape the 'radical' attenuation of language in post-minimalism. However, rather than being postmodern parody, Shea's reiteration of modernist tropes – overtly cited in the 1981 work *O Kazimir* – is a practical recourse to rediscovered formal models as a challenge to an over-determined critique of the structure, expression and ideology of the art object.

Having flirted with colour, Shea seemed to sense that outline and contour were more necessary elements in her rediscovery of language. A single work in her 1980 exhibition, *Shorts*, 1977, prefigured the development of this challenge into increasingly dimensional forms. In an anticipation of fashion's own deconstruction of boundary and surface, a pair of free-standing leather shorts explored surface texture and the relationship of interiority and exteriority through a reversal and inversion of one leg against the other – top became bottom; inside, out. Subsequent pieces became, like Maureen Connor's early

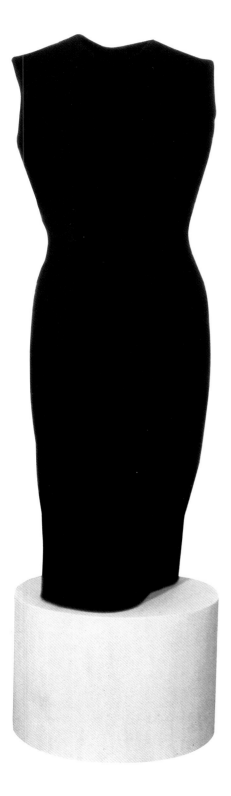

works, a means of articulating the body absent from late 1970s art through its traces, a figurative art without the figure. What became known as 'New Image' – its leading practitioners including the painter Susan Rothenberg and sculptor Joel Shapiro – was more a tendency than a fully fledged movement, but its renewed emphasis on figuration and narrative not only opened up the blind alley of language's nullification, it also paved the way for Neo-Expressionism later in the 1980s.

The stabilization of the body's trace at first took the form of a stiffening of fabric. Roughly cut felt would be soaked with colour, saturated in hot wax and then moulded around different armatures, including a male shop mannequin found in the street. A work such as *Black Dress*, 1983, has all the dimensionality, all of the expressive potential of the body it should contain, but supplemented by a certain ·pathos induced by the body's absence. Speaking of this period Shea remarked, 'I had been applying ideas from art to clothes. Clothes were basically about primary structures.... However, I began

to be interested in the idea of clothes as persons.'[6] Installed on a contrasting pedestal, *Black Dress* provoked narratives, expanded the field of meaning for its audience where post-minimalism's ideological pursuit of linguistic roots had foreclosed speculation. What is missing is the body, more commonly the subject of sculpture, more commonly read as (relatively) durable in contrast to the ephemerality of costume. The work also gives substance to that which is otherwise only flat, when hung, or, unworn, crumpled and formless on the floor. *Black Dress*, recognizably a sculpture, inverts the conventions of the mode in its choice of materials, for even if more informal substances had been pressed into service in the preceding two decades, rarely had they been used to render so overtly classical and figurative a form. This inversion is extended in the absent subject of the work and its temporality. Ostensibly a revival of classical sculpture, *Black Dress* participates in a subversion of sculpture's values even as it conforms to their pattern.

This process of inversion was simultaneously, within the oeuvre, a *retreat* from abstraction in its reach towards figuration, and, within each piece, a *working forward* from abstraction towards recognizable forms, in the shape of flat fabric cut against a clothing pattern. Shea's next step was to further challenge existing norms of sculptural practice, and at the same time undermine the representational codes of traditional sculpture. The moulded felt sculptures became another stage in the creative process, acting as the patterns for bronze and iron castings. A ceramic mould was made around the felt. In firing, this material was burned away, leaving a thin cavity that could be filled with molten metal.

Large-scale works such as *Eden*, 1986–7, and *Shield*, 1990, seem to take the artist as far from the abstractions and deliberate poverty of materials employed in post-minimalism as possible. Such a return to the forms and materials of classical sculpture might also be seen as both as ideologically conservative – a reaffirmation of traditional values that parallels the political recuperations of the Reagan era – and redundant. In the 1970s, statuary had been dismissed as monumental representations of specific ideologies, most

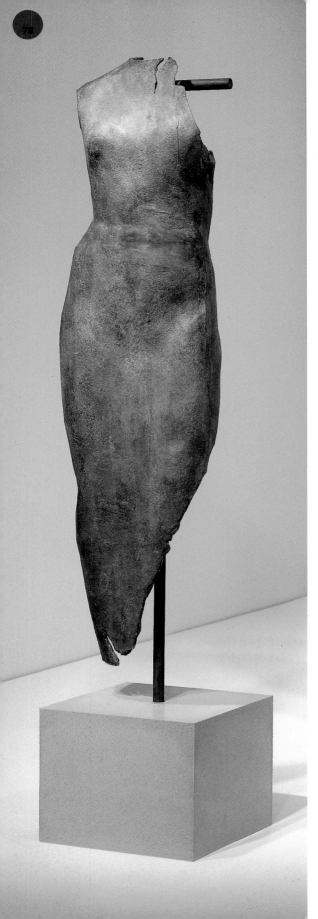

left
Judith Shea
Shield, 1990
Bronze, cast stone base

This should be silk or chiffon draped on the armature of the body, but the subject has slipped away, and the most flimsy, most fluid of materials is paradoxically fixed in the most permanent medium the artist can find.

opposite
Judith Shea
Eden, 1986–7
Bronze

A memorial to the body suffused with pathos and sense of loss. Shea's use of fashion as monumental form arrives at a figurative sculpture which is no longer heroic or erotic, but rather which mourns human ephemerality.

notably by Rosalind Krauss with her remark that 'the logic of sculpture is inseparable from the logic of the monument ... a marker at a particular place for a specific meaning/event'.[7] What such abrupt dismissals obscured, however, was the potential for critical rearticulation of a medium in its apparent obsolescence.

Shea's castings might seem to be as far from the ephemerality of fashion as they are from the non-representational strategies of the 1970s, but they use that temporal sensitivity, referenced through the non-sequiturs of a bronze coat, an iron dress, as a commentary on sculpture's apparent permanence and totality. As Peter Schjeldhal observed of Shea's work, 'Skin has no edges. Clothes do.'[8] Re-introducing a spectral figuration, Shea nonetheless, through her figuring the body out of fashion, emphasizes the edge – that totemic element of abstract sculpture – that opens the form and opens meaning. Where traditional sculpture has most often represented complete and heroic, or erotic, bodies, or their ennobled fragments, Shea inverts completion, and the relation of sculptural subject to spectator, by casting a shed skin, an absence. There ought to be bodies instead of, or at least inside of, the garments of *Eden*. Indeed the work's title evokes a relationship between nakedness and clothing, between pre-lapsarian nature and fallen culture, which leads us to suppose that these garments await still unselfconscious bodies. Shea achieves her open narratives and her critique of sculpture's completeness – which is a closure of signification as much as of the body's surface, for as Krauss rightly observed, monumentality most often signifies a historical specificity – only by a reversion to traditional materials. An interest in sculpture allows Shea to work through fashion and establish an enigma that provokes and intrigues the spectator. What we should be looking at is a pool of 'unformed' silk or cotton on the floor, almost immaterial and, slipped from the body that matters within it, almost meaningless. Fashion is, we suppose, as Hazlitt supposed, 'nothing in itself'. It needs a body in it to tell us something and then is constrained only to signify about that body, much as monument signifies event. Like the work of Connor, Benglis and others, Shea's sculpture unsettles such propositions, suggesting that the cultural structures which fashion represents may both pre-empt and perdure beyond the individual body ●

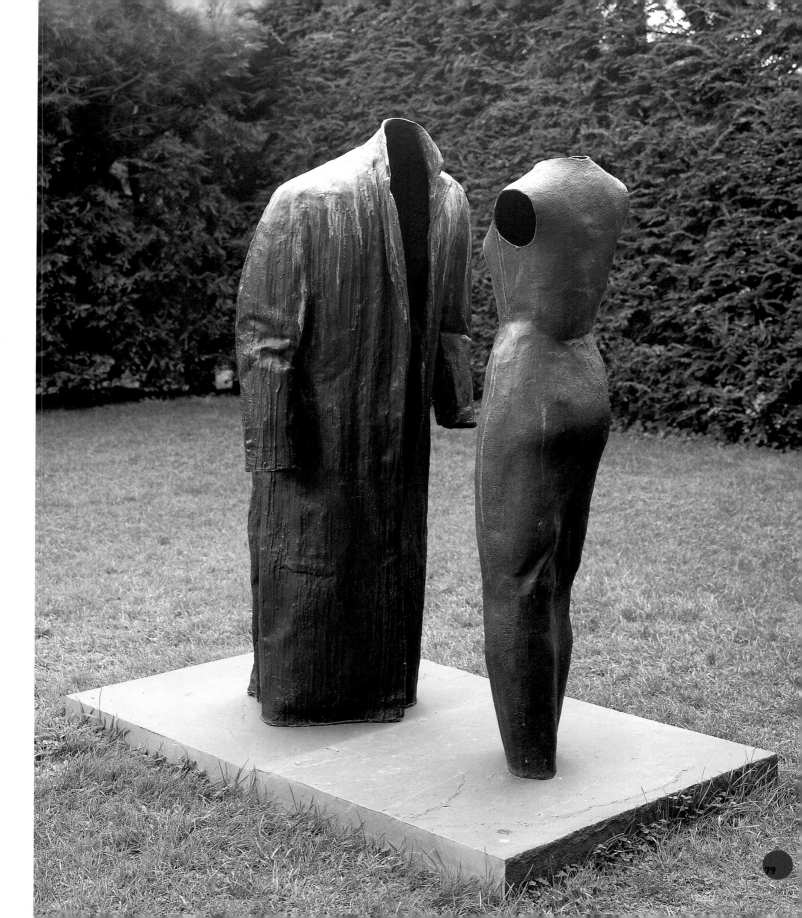

5

FRAGMENTS OF FASHION

WE HAVE ARTISTS TO TEACH US HOW TO SEE, BUT WE STILL NEED MODELS TO TEACH US HOW TO LOOK

Glenn O'Brien
Artforum

Karen Kilimnick
High Cheekbones, 1993
Acrylic and crayon on paper

The face rescued from the discarded magazine, retrieved from the fixity of photography by its transposition into a fragile, intimate medium: Kilimnick personalizes and internalizes the universal address of the fashion spread and cover shot.

Fashion changes the register of the portrait. Even the photographic study, carefully posed and lit, is imagined as limited in its circulation – if not unique – and imbued for that reason with a certain aura. The fashion magazine, with its casual, photographic proliferations, displaces the image from a solitary, painstakingly authored certainty with a specific audience into an equally authored certainty, but one with a mechanized and indifferent address. Where, painted, the image of the face might once have signified dignity, authority and respect, fashion's photograph of the face, painted or just occasionally *au naturel*, offers a wholly different set of seemingly disposable meanings. Partially obscured by blatant, competing texts, the cover model's face is presented to us in fragmentary series, a disorder of invitation. Even within the magazine, on the purer, cleaner spaces of the fashion shoot, photographic composition of the dressed body is compromised by the naming of garments. Fashion, so much, supposedly, about the look, is everywhere hemmed in by texts, and by their reading is rendered eminently forgettable. As Jeremy Gilbert-Rolfe observes, 'No one saves fashion magazines, which like fashion itself, are themselves overproductions designed to be ephemeral.'[1]

Much depends, perhaps, on what we mean by 'save'. Even the most transitory object or fleeting event may be remembered, may live in some encrypted form an after-life which requires no *obvious* physical trace. What is remembered is also 're-membered'; given a displaced, re-ordered corporeality. In *Fors*, Derrida offers a paradigm for this process, whereby what is lost is saved by its incorporation into that most obvious place of interment, the crypt. Here we have a 'saving' which simultaneously incorporates what is dead and reanimates it in obvious if encrypted physicality: for the crypt is more than a place of burial, it is also an encoding, a new way of signifying what cannot be signified. As Derrida describes the process, 'The crypt can constitute its secret only by means of its division, its fracture. "I" can save an inner safe only by putting it inside myself, *beside(s)* myself, outside.'[2] In their use of fashion imagery and symbolism, we have in two young American artists, Karen Kilimnick and T. J. Wilcox, examples of this vertiginous ambiguity: an incorporation which is simultaneously a declaration. In Kilimnick's work, in particular, we have a model for that 'I' which Derrida problematizes. Kilimnick makes 'us' of 'I'; she makes 'herself' out of what she cannot be – the image of the other, the

photographed, textually fractured, transitory fashion celebrity.

We do indeed 'save' fashion magazines. We keep them by translating their evanescence into another medium. Most often we simply wear the clothes, manifesting as exterior the interiorized identifications we have experienced in our fragmentary engagement with the fashion plate, the stylized subject of fashion. Perhaps it is no wonder that black is the staple of fashion, for all our clothes are worn in a kind of mourning for the failed, incomplete encounter with the desirable but forever intangible other. Our identity becomes a spectral re-enactment of that flawed engagement. But if our wearing fashion is an unconscious commentary on the formative processes of our own identity, artists such as Wilcox and Kilimnick – making their own investments in the processes on which they meditate – offer models of this play of loss and return in another form, specifically through the rearticulation, the encryption, of fashion's imagery.

The photograph is already a substitute for the real presence of its subject; a guarantee of presence certainly, but a translation of it into the future. Few of us will ever, unless

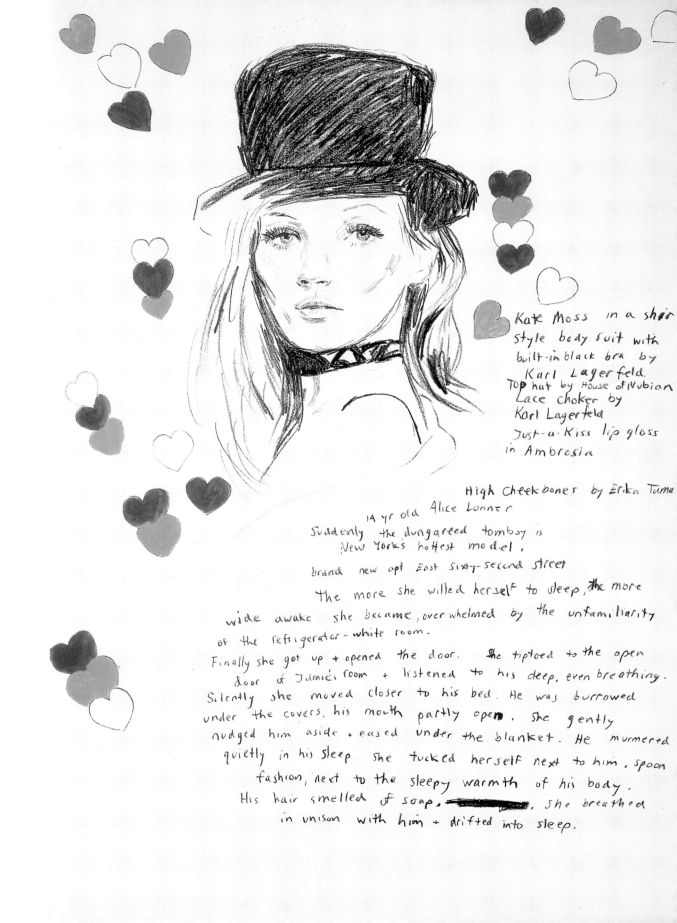

Kate Moss in a shirt
style body suit with
built-in black bra by
Karl Lagerfeld
Top hat by House of Nubian
Lace choker by
Karl Lagerfeld
Just-a-Kiss lip gloss
in Ambrosia

High cheekbones by Erika Tuma

14 yr old Alice Lonner
Suddenly the dungareed tomboy is
New York's hottest model.

brand new apt East Sixty-second Street

The more she willed herself to sleep, the more
wide awake she became, overwhelmed by the unfamiliarity
of the refrigerator-white room.
Finally she got up + opened the door. She tiptoed to the open
door of Jamie's room + listened to his deep, even breathing.
Silently she moved closer to his bed. He was burrowed
under the covers, his mouth partly open. She gently
nudged him aside + eased under the blanket. He murmered
quietly in his sleep. She tucked herself next to him, spoon
fashion, next to the sleepy warmth of his body.
His hair smelled of soap, ~~~~~~~, she breathed
in unison with him + drifted into sleep.

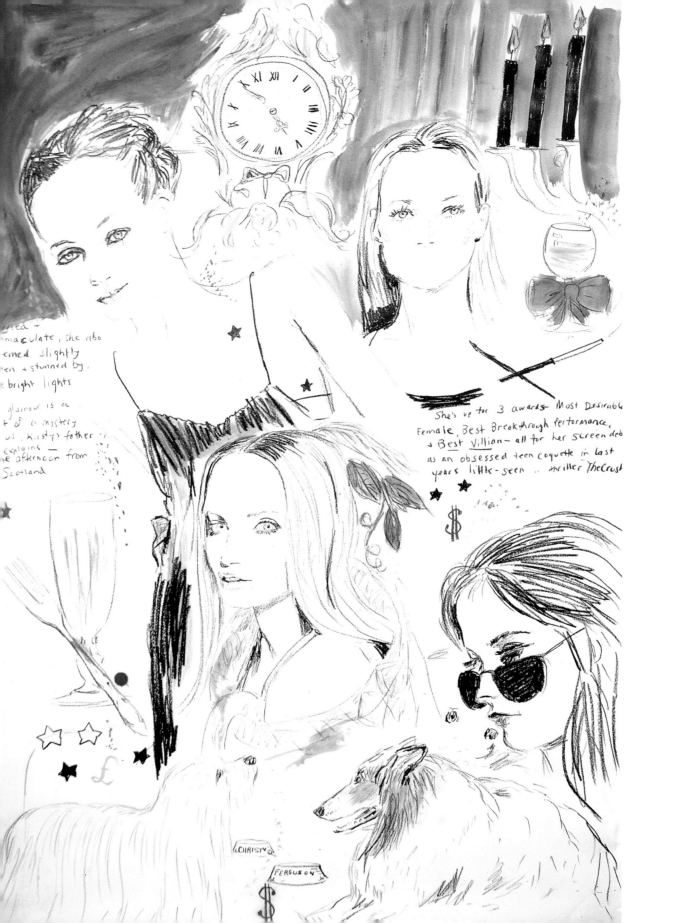

...ried - ...maculate, she also ...emed slightly ...en + stunned by. ...e bright lights

...glamour is a ...t of a mystery ...us, Kirsty's father ...explains — ...e afternoon from Scotland

She's up for 3 awards: Most Desirable Female, Best Breakthrough Performance, & Best Villian - all for her screen debut as an obsessed teen coquette in last years little-seen .. thriller TheCrush

CHRISTY
FERGUSON
$

Karen Kilimnick
Curried and Immaculate, 1994
Acrylic, crayon and pastel on paper

'I am you, and I want to be you –
all of you.' Kilimnick's drawings look
like the project of an obsessed fan
who, in her head, shares the lives of
top models. The drawings illustrate
how fashion shapes our desires.

very privileged, see Amber Valletta wearing Versace as she does for Steven Meisel, see Stella Tennant stroll down a catwalk for Helmut Lang. Even in its most joyous, most erotic address, the photograph is permeated by melancholy, for it is both the manifestation of the intangible, and simultaneously, always, the space of time past, of that which has been. As the French critic Christian Metz writes, 'Even when the person photographed is still living, that moment when he or she was has forever vanished. Strictly speaking, the person *who has been photographed* – not the total person, who is an effect of time – is dead: dead for having been seen.'[3] The fashion photograph initiates an imaginary relationship with a carefully constructed, already vanished subject. Once that relationship is established, it matters little what happens to the picture. The medium becomes immaterial. It is our picture of the image that we carry around with us, folding it into the perpetually shifting sets of desires and imaginations that we call our selves. When Derrida problematizes 'I' and 'myself', he is drawing attention precisely to the constitution of the terms of identity through incorporation of others. 'We' do not have an exterior reference point from which to contemplate the process of our being.

Karen Kilimnick renders explicit this never-completed sum of identifications and desires. Her drawings are often based upon the pervasive fashion photograph, but they displace its register once again, back into the unique and the hand-crafted. Kilimnick's media are, however, light and informal: crayon, pastel and ink, rather than paints or even artist's crayon. These are at once the materials of provisionality – the media of the study, the preparation for the more important work – and the materials of childhood art. Kilimnick's drawings are a self-consciously diminished practice, a minor art which demonstrates that we never complete the bigger picture. These sketches look like the work of an infatuated teenager, a conception reinforced by the artist's occasional recourse to glitter, magic marker and fake plastic jewelry to elaborate the image. Through a faux-intimacy with her subjects, Kilimnick does occupy the shoes of the young girl who wants to be a supermodel, but she is also the woman who desires elegance and luxury rather than quotidian routine: in other words, the average reader of the fashion magazine. By a conscious assumption of these roles – admitting that they might, too, be a part of her identity, and that the artworks which depict them might not, then, be the products of detached, objective consciousness – Kilimnick illustrates fashion's fashioning of our identities.

In the fragmentary, contested solicitation of the model's face, she becomes both the object we desire – what we want to possess – and the object with which we identify – the possessor of attributes that we might also want to own. The latter imagination compensates us for the impossibility of desire. Unable to take hold of what is lost to us, we instead take it as our role model. When Derrida refers to the crypt as 'the vault of a desire'[4] he rightly divines identity as the interment of habitual failure. We *never* get what we want. Despite the glamour that Kilimnick simultaneously vitiates and exaggerates, the process of identification she represents is, as Diana Fuss puts it 'an embarrassingly ordinary process, a routine, habitual recompense for the everyday loss of our love objects'.[5] If, as Freud suggests,[6] identification is a process of unconsciously selecting ideals, then perhaps that recognition of ideality only emerges through the displacement of desire, its translation into another register. The incorporation of loss into the self is central to Freud's commentary in his essay 'Mourning and Melancholia'[7] and we might understand through it that, if the subject of any photograph is already 'dead', lost in the moment of our first encounter, then our engagement with the fashion model is both suffused with pleasure, and profoundly, if unconsciously, traumatic, because desire is simultaneous with its frustration.

What is lost in fashion is something over which, properly speaking, we've never really

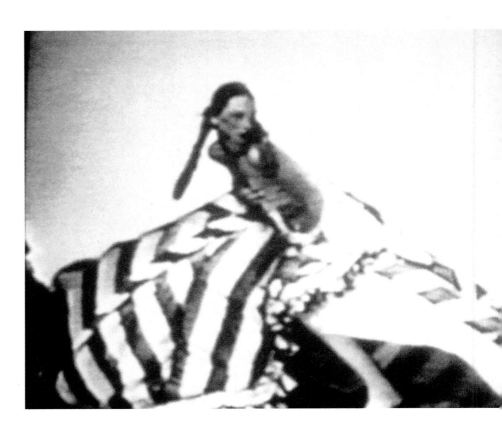

had discretionary rights. Our identities, meanwhile, become palimpsests of compensation. We are what we cannot be; what we cannot grasp; what our hands pass through. Such is the condition of the obsessive, but Kilimnick makes it transparently clear that this consuming, unsustainable longing permeates our identity beyond the limits of safely pathologized categories. We are all obsessives: the fashion and celebrity industries make us so, and we manufacture fashion and celebrity to (almost) sate our continual demands. All our identities are built on these continual encounters. We 'save' images; we even, in a way, 'save' fashion magazines.

Jacques Lacan suggests a certain affinity for this process of incorporating the other to both the photograph and the treasured object, faded, folded, kept, that substitutes for experience. 'What one cannot keep outside one always keeps as an image within. Identification with the object of love is as stupid as that.'[8] But if what we are is determined by slipping an imaginary image of the other into the folds of our clothing and the corrugations of our identity, this burial of the 'dead' also takes other forms of

encryption. Those folds are themselves a kind of story, another text about someone else through which we are becoming ourselves. We codify this incorporative process; we invent narrative. It is through narrative that fashion photography seduces us, invites us to participate in its scenarios. 'Hey mister, that's me up there, on the balcony, the castle walls, in Saint Laurent or Gucci; on the beach, in the surf, in Dolce & Gabbana; in a crack-den basement, opiate thin, in whatever's appropriate to the narcotic moment.' And it is this insertion of the self into the context of the other – in the form of the other – that is at the heart of Kilimnick's fashion drawings. Kate, Naomi, Amber and Cindy are her friends. In *What Time Should We Leave?*, 1995, they hang out together in the Hamptons, endlessly discussing designers, make-up, model agency politics, luxury hotels and first-class air travel. This is not only art making explicit the solicitations of fashion, the beckoning gestures of revenants, it is art making plain the mechanics of identity formation and revelling in their complexity, their fragmentation, their continual incompletion.

In a Kilimnick drawing nothing ever quite adds up. Text frames and displaces image in

the same moment as it complements it. Where fashion's text explains – what it is, where to buy it – Kilimnick's offers hand-crafted histories, marginal testimonies from unnamed protagonists which may often have only a tangential bearing on the subject of her drawing, and which excavate fashion's own deep-buried traumas, the petty jealousies and misplaced affections, the addictions, deaths and doppelgangers. *I'm not who you think I am, and I hate you too*, 1994, has a half-naked model, a mask slipped from her eyes over her mouth, return the artist's gaze. For Kilimnick this image is unusually direct: a picture that explains the mute performance of identity within fashion, and that, by 'speaking' through the text, ruptures its façade to reveal our greatest fear – that what we love is not only false, but that it despises us. If we are the never-completed sum of our identifications – that continual accretion of identity mirrored in the acquisition of new garments – then, Kilimnick suggests, bracketed somewhere in that equation is the turning of the other's hatred onto, into, our selves.

The hatred of the dead: a small price to pay for our seduction by fashion and its models.

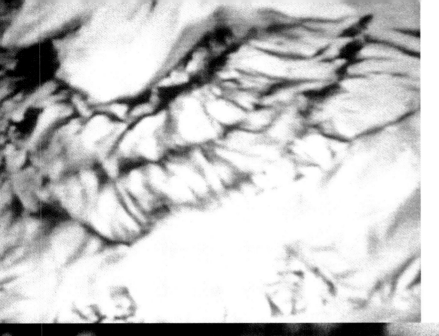

T. J. Wilcox
Photographs from the film
*The Escape (of Marie Antoinette),
Nos. 2, 3 and 6*, 1996
C print and R prints

Fragments of Galliano's dream
of elegance, imported into a
whimsical narrative of identity
and excess. Contemporary fashion
becomes a signifier for frivolity
and ephemerality in history.

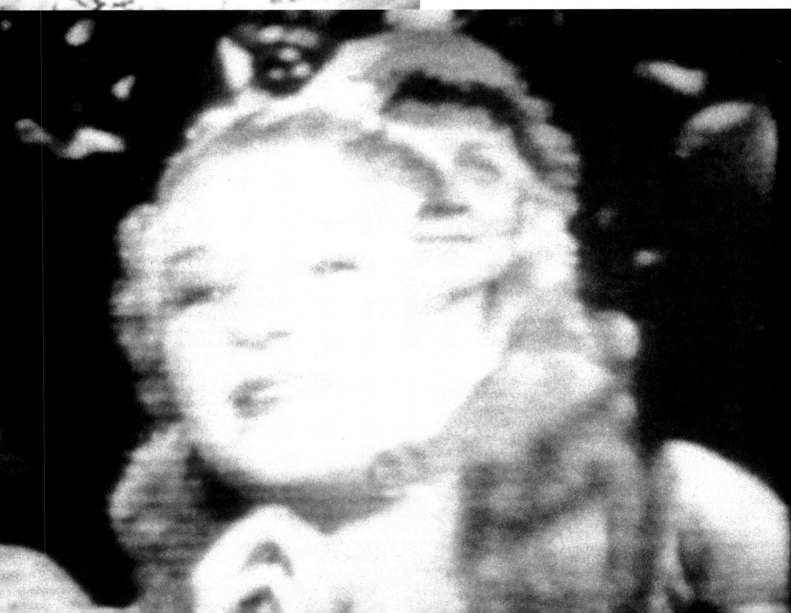

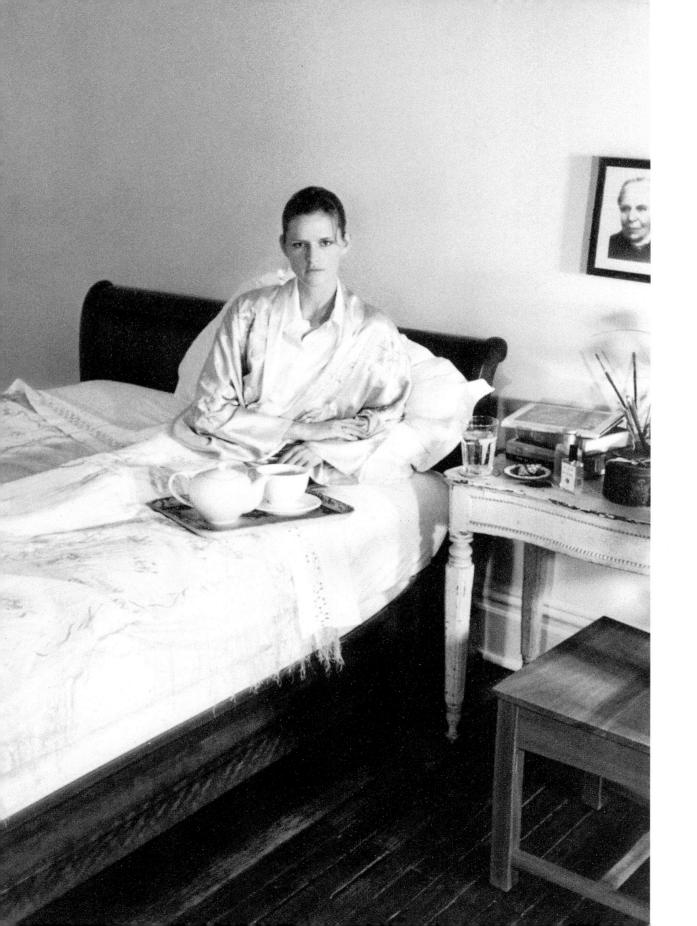

T. J. Wilcox
Stephen Tennant Hommage, No. 6, 1997
R print

If Stella Tennant plays her wonderfully
decadent ancestor, the dilettante
writer Stephen Tennant, then T. J.
Wilcox becomes Cecil Beaton, the
master fashion photographer. It is not
only genders that are inverted here.
Art and fashion combine to pastiche
the historical relationship of fashion
and art.

As if the photograph, always a revenant, was not trauma enough. Perhaps that is why Kilimnick's fragmentary, cryptic narratives are not themselves photographic. To address the loss of the object and, in its evanescence, the object's slight to our longing, she changes media and translates death into a language which can be borne. Fashion photography is, even when it's fun, a serious business: witness the po-faced faux-cruelty of Helmut Newton, often as repetitive and dull as a de Sade novel. Kilimnick's adaptations resort to whimsy – we might even call them fey – but their retreat from the obsessive self-importance of the fashion plate also opens a perspective on the past, on fashion's failed promise, its 'always was', that the immediacy of the photograph, its 'always now', elides. There's a certain deliberate archaism about this recourse to drawing: who now pays fashion illustrators?

There's a certain archaism, and a similar whimsicality, too, about T. J. Wilcox's sense of fashion, its footage not so seamlessly incorporated into his films. There is also, in the compositional process, a series of complex transactions between film and video and film. Wilcox's work flickers and jumps before our eyes like the spectacle of early cinema, its 16mm film an antiquated gauge, the fragile projector rattling as it unrolls the artist's collaged vision. Everything that Wilcox uses is first filmed in Super-8 – a medium as delicate, democratic and transitory as Kilimnick's crayons; its colours unstable, its spooling hesitant, its perspective fixed. What Wilcox films may itself already be film or video – as with the footage of a John Galliano catwalk show in *The Escape (of Marie Antoinette)*, 1996. The Super-8 film is transferred to video for editing, and then to 16mm film for projection. With each change of medium there is a loss of image from the original, but simultaneously a novel and unique identity emerges. Wilcox's filmic process seems to mimic the unconscious transactions we undertake with images: incorporating, translating, folding into ourselves. As Wilcox himself observes, 'At the labs they always think I'm losing image, but I always feel like I'm getting something new with each step in the process. I became interested in this accumulating aspect of the process and this surplus of work that had a spectacular beauty as its result.'[9]

Wilcox takes as his subjects individuals who used fashion as part of a strategy of 'self-fashioning', a partially conscious construction of the self in the social world. The central characters in films such as *Stephen Tennant Hommage* and *The Escape (of Marie Antoinette)* hyperbolize their identity through excess, whether of clothing, financial extravagance or behaviour. These are lives 'devoted to the ephemeral', as Wilcox says of Tennant, emphasizing the connections by having the model Stella Tennant play the role of her ancestor.[10] Even in a more recent film, a charming version of Babar the Elephant, the little elephant's entry into society is only effected when a wealthy lady buys him a suit. The frivolous and the transitory become vital elements in a strikingly artificial architecture of identity. These are indeed spectacularly artificial individuals, their lives shaped by costume changes and magpie appropriations, but the trajectories of their futility also, in their histories, in their exaggeration, are the trajectories of our own engagements with the world writ large. Fashion, as much a crypt as our unconscious, contains and conceals our bodies and flaunts both corporeality and 'true' identity. Wilcox and Kilimnick's works themselves operate through forms of encryption – Wilcox by translating between media and by 'burying' clips of footage within his films, Kilimnick through an exchange between the photograph and the drawing, between the immediacy of experience and the return of its metamorphosed form in memory. Both use an engagement with fashion to make clear, and perhaps to celebrate, its complicity in our being who we are ●

6

SHOPPING IN SPACE

IT'S VERY FANCY ON OLD DELANCEY STREET, YOU KNOW

Richard Rogers and Lorenz Hart
'Manhattan' from *The Garrick Gaieties*, 1925

SoHo had been one thing – a vibrant community of avant-garde artists in cheap lofts. Now it was another. Fashion had been one thing – an imaginary pastiche of history and oriental culture, remote from the radical culture of its time. Now it was another – in SoHo. In a district of Manhattan which had, for twenty years, played host to much of the New York avant-garde's most innovative activity, a divide came down: time was embodied in the allure of shop fronts, disembodied in the evanescence and adumbration of halogen-spot-lit spaces, embodied in the attitudes of retail assistants and their customers. What had seemed like a stable community was disrupted by the growing number of new arrivals – commercial stores, many of them purveying high fashion. Galleries moved off the street, as artists moved out of lofts they'd bought cheap or let illegally, so rates rose for the strangers who moved in, strangers who were, perhaps, collectors, but not often creators. The editors of the radical arts journal *October*, some of them SoHo dwellers, saw this process – the erosion of the geographical and social space of 'their' avant-garde – as 'the brute logic of the market economy'.[1] They contrasted the assumed purity and originality of their generation's vanguard artists with the apparently market-driven complicity of the next, at that time caught up in an earlier phase of gentrification's cycle half a dozen blocks away in the East Village.[2] This critique neglected to mention that the very conditions for SoHo's foundation as fine-art community – including the gentrification of Greenwich Village – were themselves established in the same economy which, from the mid-1980s, overwhelmed SoHo and propagated studio spaces and new galleries over on Avenue C.

Since, in combination with its relatively low rents, SoHo's very status as avant-garde community, almost regardless of the style of art it produced, had been in part the attraction for a new generation of retailers, fashion ingratiated itself by collaborating on art projects and displayed its own good taste, its creativity and its recognition of other's particular visions. Fashion also displayed its commercial power, its disruptive effect and its very different sense of history. Even as these projects legitimated fashion's entry into the space of art – into its studios, cafés, its community, rather than the concepts it had for some time cohabited – they offered a site for critiques, and even outright rejections, which could discomfit the business sense that all was well with the world.

'Fashion' was not some disembodied entity: such projects gave it names and presence. Recognition of the name – the brand – was after all a significant motive for these collaborations. The fashion retailer Comme des Garçons, which had arrived on Wooster Street as early as 1982, involved itself in 'Architectures of Display'. Organized by the Architectural League of New York, with the local architectural project Minetta Brook, this series of installations addressed the relationship of structure and spectacle in contemporary and historical terms. The critic Reinhold Martin described the issues that the project raised in the process of its development. 'To what extent do terms and conventions of display affect definitions of "public space"? What kinds of intersubjective relations are set up in instances of display? What are their effects?'[3] *Like the Difference between Autumn/Winter '94/'95 and Spring/Summer '95*, installed in the Comme des Garçons store by artist Silvia Kolbowski

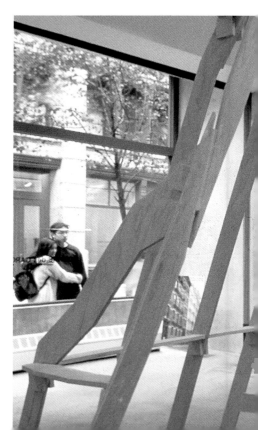

Silvia Kolbowski and Peter Eisenman
Like the Difference between Autumn/Winter '94/'95 and Spring/Summer '95, 1995, installed in Comme des Garçons store, Wooster Street, New York
Mixed media and conceptual diagrams

The awkwardness of art's accommodation with fashion made palpable. Kolbowski and Eisenman used fashion's money and fashion's space to provoke discussion about the fundamental changes in an area – SoHo – that had been home to the avant-garde for nearly twenty years.

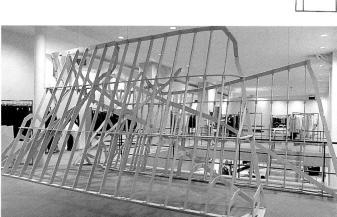

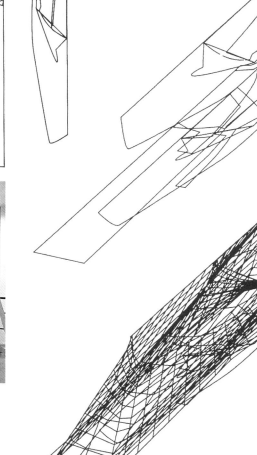

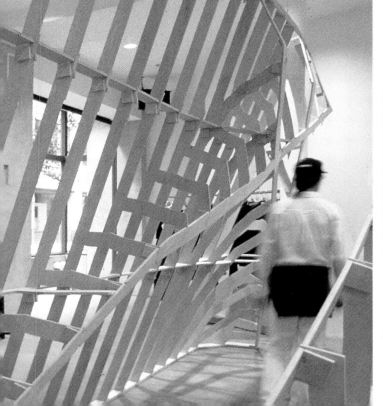

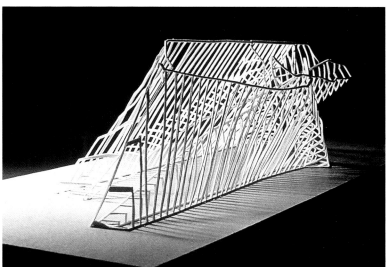

with the architect Peter Eisenman, seemed to raise other questions beyond those identified by Martin. Their interrogation did not provide the safe answers, the accommodation within community, that Comme des Garçons perhaps sought. Rather, *Like the Difference between Autumn/Winter '94/'95 and Spring/Summer '95* seemed to emphasize resistance and loss, encapsulating the schism between two radically distinct perceptions, not necessarily of the object, but of time and memory.

Martin went on to identify the following 'Site Conditions':

1 a 'high' fashion store in a 'high' art neighborhood.
2 the 'newness' of seasonal fashion in a bell jar neighborhood (SoHo).
3 glass as a membrane between perpetual change and preservation.
4 a late 20th-century shift from shallow storefront display housing object narratives to transparency and non narrativity.
5 a historical change from lateral scenography to a depth of field scenario.
6 the intervention of fine art into a commercial art site.
7 objects on display for sale (window dressing) and objects on display ('just looking').[4]

The response to these conditions was a barrier, a 'wall', dividing the space of fashion's commerce from the street, but also from the community – the space and structure into which it had intruded. The wall in Wooster Street embodied both Kolbowski and Eisenman's, and Comme des Garçons founder Rei Kawakubo's preoccupations with a different sense of structure: preoccupations which acknowledged

and emphasized the body rather than overwhelmed it and also reflected the artists' commitment to memory. Eisenman had founded his reputation on formal challenges to the dimensional constants of Western architectural history – the vertical and the horizontal. His buildings deconstructed conventional relationships and instead emphasized the folded, the offset, the disjunctive. A similar challenge had been presented to the formal structures of fashion by Kawakubo since the first exhibitions of her work on a catwalk. The intervention in Comme des Garçons' space would be premised upon a resistance to forgetting, to a mnemonic continuity rather than a sense of the past punctuated by elision and abrupt recollection. Kolbowski devised a concept for the project whereby the shape of the wall was derived from a palimpsest of Comme des Garçons design sketches, taken from the seasons autumn/winter 1994/1995 and spring/summer 1995. Kolbowski and Eisenman then morphed these outlines by computer to generate an incidental form whose structural elements paraphrased the physical differences between the two design projects. Since the earlier of these collections was now history – obsolete clothing no longer acknowledged by commerce – Kolbowski and Eisenman's structure embodied a memory that fashion did not want to have, stressing continuity over rupture and reintroducing what had recently been alienated.

This wall, however, was not a wall. Certainly it served as a barrier: indeed, its very permeability, canted members and skeletal openness, the very fact that it worked also as a conduit, emphasized its awkwardness and resistance to the space it inhabited. A white wall, perpendicular to the floor, would have conformed, even as a barrier, to the demands

of the existing space. Such a structure might have represented a contribution from art, a structural element of the 'white cube' of minimalist, modernist exhibition, but that was the state to which the Comme des Garçons store already aspired. This was a wall you could – indeed, had to – walk through: only ghosts, only memories, got to walk through walls. Rather than being 'a wall', Kolbowski and Eisenman's construction made plain the structure of a wall – a deconstruction of architecture which worked in the same way as Kawakubo's clothes, similarly retaining use value, similarly highlighting their presence. By installing temporality as a fundamental of the structure, the artists deployed those shared 'deconstructive' precepts against fashion. The insistence on memory rebuked fashion's forgetfulness of its own past and, at the same time, memorialized SoHo's artistic history and community, now threatened with erasure in the district's reconfiguration as commercial space. The 'wall' forms the egress for the Comme des Garçons store behind it, but whilst it obstructed the spectatorial gaze from the street – both soliciting and resisting those who were 'just looking' – in addition it transformed the retail space to which it became threshold. We might, returning again to Derrida's concept of *Fors*, say that Kolbowski and Eisenman encrypted that space. Their structure changed its meaning, encoding it, and buried it in an obvious entombment, behind the means of its access, a narrow and easily obstructed passage.

Comme des Garçons' patronage of this confrontation to, and hampering of, its presence, made a strange kind of sense – even though the company's reception of Kolbowski and Eisenman's project was

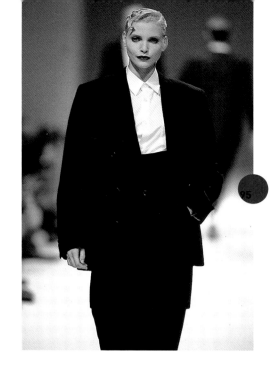

clockwise from top right
Comme des Garçons
suit, spring/summer 1995; suit with
full skirt, spring/summer 1995;
cap-sleeved asymmetric coat-dress,
autumn/winter 1994/95; long dress,
autumn/winter 1994/95

For the artist (Kolbowski), the
architect (Eisenman) and the fashion
designer (Kawakubo), there is a
shared preoccupation with a particular
sense of structure. All seem to want
an architecture that emphasizes
rather than overwhelms the body.

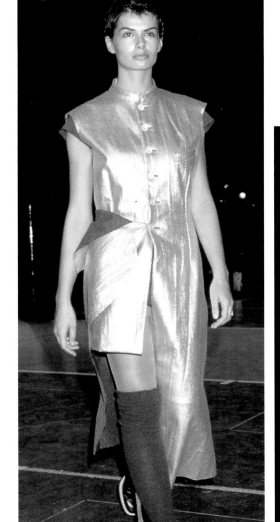

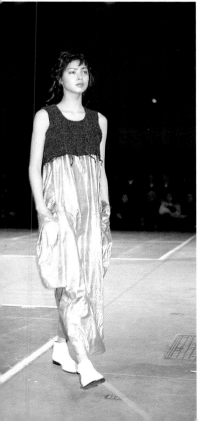

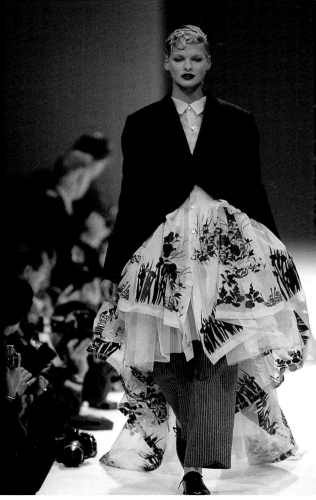

increasingly chilly. By 1995 bringing art into the retail space was a well-established strategy for fashion stores seeking to enhance their cultural profile. Although Ingrid Sischy had recently announced in *The New Yorker* that fashion had replaced art as the centre of cultural attention, in their recourse to art as (unsaleable) object it seemed as though the retailers did not yet quite believe in that shift. The low-scale collaborations typified by Cindy Sherman's 'Dianne B' photographs had, throughout the 1980s and early '90s, escalated into major projects of donation, sponsorship and partnership, and despite its evident lack of sympathy to its patrons, *Like the Difference between Autumn/Winter '94/'95 and Spring/Summer '95* must be understood in this context.

For his 1993 exhibition 'Skins', at the Grey Art Gallery, the French artist Gotscho had deployed thirty Agnès b jackets, in addition to Hermès saddle bags and various items by Gianfranco Ferre. These works, combining elegant furniture with high fashion, invoked a profound pathos for the absent body – specifically, for those cognisant with Gotscho's biography, the body absented through AIDS – and its inadequate substitution by the commodity. Agnès b had been a prominent figure in the convergence of art and fashion over the previous decade, exhibiting works by Sherman and Robert Mapplethorpe, amongst others, in-store, and using their images in corporate advertising. Helmut Lang would follow suit, installing a recently acquired neon by Jenny Holzer in his Greene Street store, and embarking on a series of minimalist advertisements, often placed in art magazines, each of which contained an iconic contemporary artwork. In London's Covent Garden, if you entered

one of the downstairs changing rooms in Paul Smith's menswear store, you could find, discreetly tucked away in a corner, Euan Uglow's *La Bapistry Castiglione Olana* (sic): art to contemplate while you tried on your new suit. Meanwhile, Comme des Garçons, who would also work with the greatly-in-demand Cindy Sherman both in its Tokyo Aoyama store and in corporate advertising, produced an in-house magazine, *Sixth Sense*, whose content and production values challenged the boundaries between art and fashion journals. Writing on Comme des Garçons and its relationship to the art world in the late 1980s, critic Glenn O'Brien remarked, 'The clothing it manufactures and markets is like art in every respect except being art. And now it has created one of the great art magazines of our time, except that it's not really an art magazine, it's a clothing catalogue.'[5]

Many of the exchanges between artists and designers were driven along by close friendships, often formed prior to the projects, though in some cases initiating them, and in others developing through them. This was not, of course, a wholly novel state of affairs: the couturier Paul Poiret, for example, had been unstinting in his support for Dufy and Man Ray in the 1920s, and British fashion retailer Selfridges had shown contemporary artists' work, including Henry Moore's, in-store during the 1930s. The friendship between the star painter of the '80s, Julian Schnabel, and fashion designer Azzedine Alaïa, which led to Schnabel undertaking interior designs for Alaïa's workshop, and Alaïa making clothes for Schnabel's friends, can be understood as echoing such relationships. The fraternity of artists and fashion's producers would resonate further in the new century with such concords as the

friendships of Tracey Emin and Vivienne Westwood, or Sam Taylor-Wood with Joseph Corré and Serena Rees, founders of Agent Provocateur. For Christmas 2001 Corré and Rees's company would supply the shop at Tate Modern with a range of exclusive lingerie.

By the late 1990s, however, the engagement of corporate fashion with art projects would attain a new prominence, both in terms of sponsorship and in the novel strategy of companies founding their own art museums. Paul Smith, as an iconic figure in British fashion and acknowledged master of branding, worked with Tate Modern to design the uniforms for guards in the rebranding of a national institution. In April 1998, Gucci, its tired profile radically transformed under the aegis of young American designer Tom Ford, and by now part of the Pinault-Printemps-Redoute retail group (a luxury brands conglomerate which would shortly acquire the prestigious Christie's auction house) supported *Show*, the most significant performance to that date by the young American artist Vanessa Beecroft. If Smith was 'dressing the museum', Beecroft and Ford 'undressed' it. In the central cockpit of New York's Guggenheim, Beecroft arrayed twenty fashion models, dressed at most in Gucci heels, thongs and tops, with some wearing considerably less. The models stood or, when tired, sat, in public scrutiny, fixedly returning the gazes that were trained upon them. At one level looking like a tableau vivant of Helmut Newton's wildest fantasies, the apparently vulnerable models exuded only an uncanny blankness contaminated perhaps by a certain potential for violence. The eroticism that is fashion's veiled subject was made literal in palpable, and somewhat bored, flesh. The body as object of

Vanessa Beecroft
Show, 2001
Performance

Beecroft turns the fashion photograph
into a tableau. You might say 'tableau
vivant' if the poses weren't so static.
Wearing Gucci, when they wear
anything, the regimented models
are at once a wild sexual fantasy
and its dissipation.

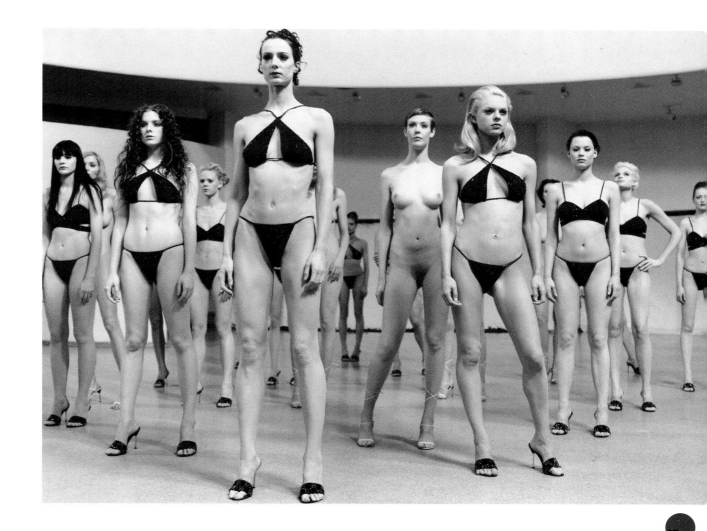

prolonged contemplation returned that gaze with interest, and the consequences for the viewer were potentially discomfiting. Unlike a Newton photograph, say *Sie Kommen*, 1981, this was no passive spectacle of femininity's threat – though the photographs that Beecroft took to document the performance made it into one. Through the flesh, Beecroft could be understood to directly invert the visual regime that structures a fashion photograph, whilst insisting precisely on the coldness and cruelty of Newton's subjects. Gucci's material contribution to this hyperbolization and inversion of body and gaze was itself a hyperbolization of the relationships which had preceded it. However, like the development of patronage and collaboration, Beecroft's Guggenheim extravaganza occupies a historical continuum, an evolution of supportive relationships that runs from such involvements as Schiaparelli's costuming of films by Man Ray, and Buñuel and Dalí, and her provision of mannequins for the 1938 Surrealist exhibition in Paris.

For fashion houses to fund their own museums was a new step, beyond the traditional patronage of endowments and gifts to established institutions. Pursued by both Prada, with Fondazione Prada in Milan, and Cartier, with Fondation Cartier pour l'Art Contemporain in Paris, such a policy established a far higher public profile for corporate identity than either endowment or sponsorship. However, these commitments by well-established fashion brands seem to go beyond promotional exercises. Rather, they reflect a profound faith on the part of boards and individuals in the creative processes and values of art. Some corporations, for example Selfridges – reviving the company's pre-war interest

Sam Taylor-Wood
XV Seconds, June-October 2000
Installation of photographs on the façade of Selfridges, London

Continuing the store's seventy-year tradition of exhibiting the avant-garde, and emphasizing hip cultural credentials in a reshaped marketing profile, Taylor-Wood freezes the celebrity and the model as art rather than advertising.

below
Jean Nouvel (architect)
Fondation Cartier pour l'art contemporain, Paris

Instead of patronage and endorsement – the traditional relationship of enterprise to public culture – the corporation simply founds its own museum.

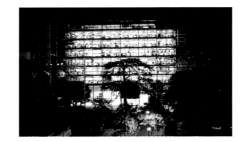

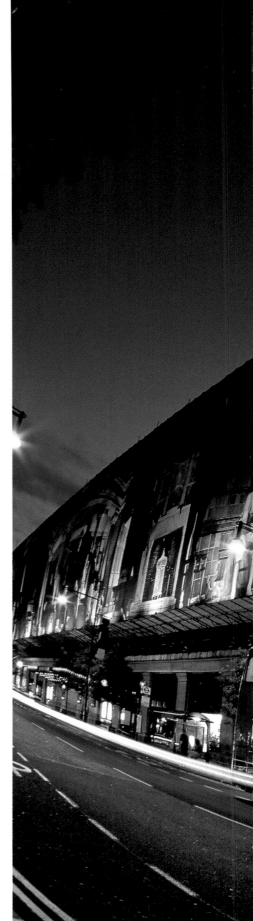

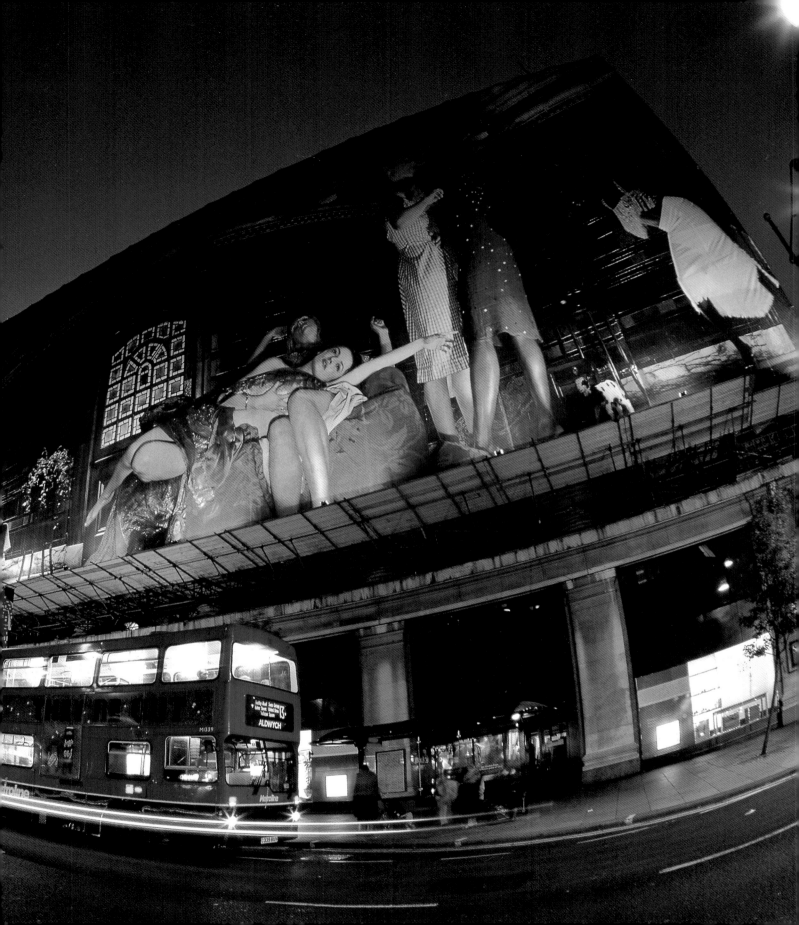

in art – had undertaken regular programmes of high-profile exhibition and commission that, in the opinion of the company's directors, were at least as effective in commercial terms as other aspects of its marketing and advertising spend.[6] However, whilst there might be a commercially useful strand to the enterprise of the corporate museum, such projects depend ultimately on the same enthusiasms that founded public collections and museums across Europe and North America earlier in the nineteenth and twentieth centuries.

Like the Difference between Autumn/Winter '94/'95 and Spring/Summer '95 was not, however, an isolated example of resistance to, and critique of, this accelerating and mutually enchanted convergence. Sue Coe's 'Sweat Shop' series of 1994 consisted of drawings, watercolours and gouaches which drew attention to the plight of under-paid, under-aged, under-represented workers in the Third World, producing fashion garments for major international corporations. Coe's work came at much the same time as the first campaigns drawing attention to this egregious exploitation. Elsewhere the challenge to fashion surfaced in more ironic but nonetheless effective projects such as that of Art Club 2000, a group of seven young artists whose 'Commingle' exhibition of 1993 had included photographs of group members dressed entirely in Gap clothing, 'borrowed' Gap display materials and stencilled quotations from Gap internal staff directives and literature. Art Club 2000 had also applied for jobs at Gap and documented the garbage thrown out at various Gap stores across Manhattan. As Glenn O'Brien remarked, 'If artists aren't going to make

fun of artily positioned institutions, who's going to do it?'[7] This ironic and appropriative assault upon the fashion corporation would reach its apotheosis in an infamous (and one might say brilliant) spoof advertisement by the *Los Angeles Times* magazine, affirming that, like a great many other luminaries honoured by Gap at that time, Hitler too wore khakis.

In a text for a 1997 project that examined the relocation of galleries from SoHo to Chelsea, Silvia Kolbowski would describe a dream. 'As I travel floor to floor I notice that some of the enterprises are just finishing elegant renovations, but I can't tell whether the spaces are being renovated to hold clothing stores or galleries. Due to the fact that I'm being rushed out of these spaces by not-overly-friendly staff, it is particularly difficult to discern the differences, although I do now remember that one of the spaces, significantly on an upper floor, was selling clothing, and I was standing at a counter that had the minimal look of a gallery desk, but at which one could purchase something.'[8] If Kolbowski's dream reflected an anxiety about the convergence of art and fashion to the point where gallery and store were indistinguishable, she had already provided a similarly oneiric motif for this intersection in a contribution to *Like the Difference between Autumn/Winter '94/'95 and Spring/Summer '95*. Kolbowski and Eisenman's installation (see p. 12) mimed the retailer's practice of including a video of catwalk display within their specially created environment. This footage shared the technique of morphing together the two collections, old and new, which had been used in the wall. In the video there is the temporal simultaneity which

characterizes events in a dream. Everyone is spectral and immediate, their figures passing through each other, converging, intersecting and re-emerging. Here past haunts present, present haunts past, and the present haunts itself. Only an expert on the two collections could discern which time is which. Where the architectural form incorporated the linear range of memory and extended it as structure, here it is compressed into the condition of the photograph, where all moments of time past exist in time present. *Like the Difference between Autumn/Winter '94/'95 and Spring/Summer '95* reflected a fundamental difference in the temporalities of art and fashion: where art insists on the continued value of object (and concept) beyond its moment of production and immediate reception (give or take a few years of neglect to compensate for any immediate fashionability of presentation), fashion's time is intermittent, seasonal and circular.

Even if fashion's formal and narrative structures represented a recourse for art that took it from self-scrutiny back to rhetoric, this difference would eventually prove a significant stumbling block in aesthetic, if not economic, convergence. In the work of young artists, only a few years after Kolbowski and Eisenman's project, a dissatisfaction with the temporality of fashion's objects would be articulated in violence against them. In the patterns of Kolbowski's 'ghosts' on screen, their crossing and recrossing, the vision of one time, one body, walking out of another, we might recognize a certain symbolization of art and fashion's intersection, and with it a dream-like anticipation that one might pass, forever, through the other to once more occupy a separate domain ●

right
Art Club 2000
Untitled (Times Square/Gap Grunge 2),
1992–3
C print

below
Art Club 2000
Untitled (Conran's 1), 1992–3
C print

Ironizing the pervasiveness
and ubiquity of the supposedly hip
and exclusive brand, and parodying
the reality of the perfect life
portrayed in advertising, Art Club
2000 remodels Gap.

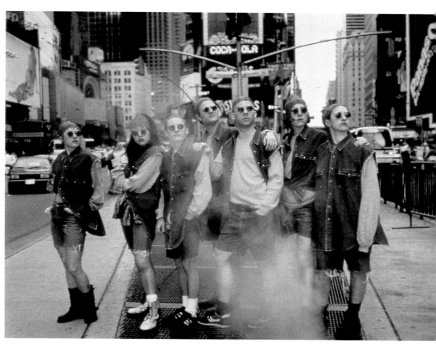

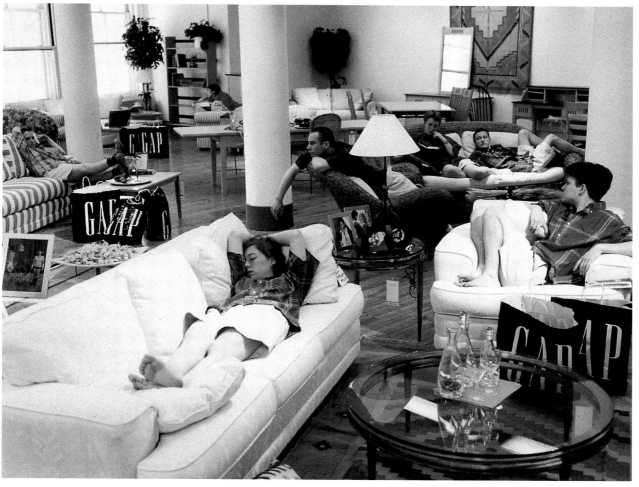

FORM AND UNIFORM

TED: I CAN'T BELIEVE YOU'RE WEARING THAT UNIFORM. ARE YOU OUT OF YOUR MIND?

FRED: THIS IS THE CORRECT UNIFORM

Whit Stillman,
screenplay for *Barcelona*, 1992

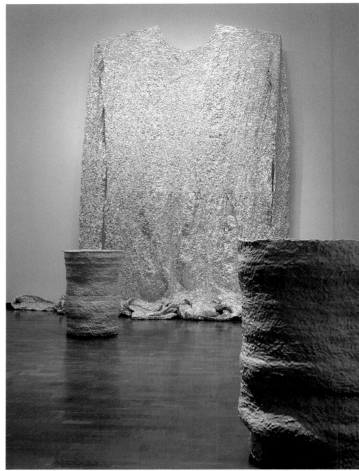

right
Beverly Semmes
Big Silver, 1996
Lamé cloth, motor, hardware

A convergence of fashion and
the dancer's body, endlessly
repeating its manoeuvres, Semmes's
work entertains us by continually
shifting its position. The sculpture
continues the dance by other means,
beyond the limits of its space.

below
Beverly Semmes
Red Dress, 1992
Velvet, wood, metal hanger

An almost preposterous grandiosity
of the body, its impossible scale
deflated by 'normal' arms; a 'dress'
formally stunning in its colour and
shape, which nonetheless invites us
to compose our own narratives about
what kind of body might inhabit it.

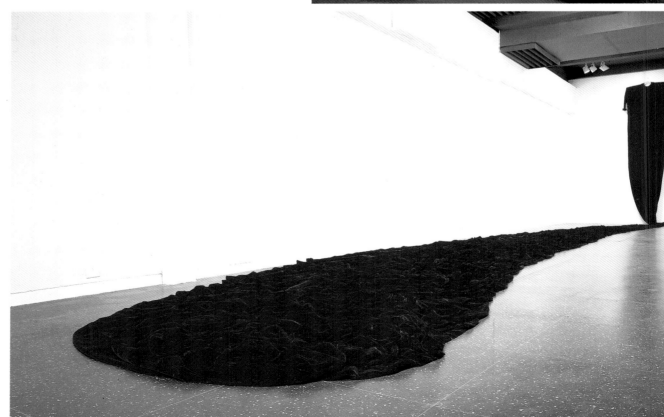

below left
Beverly Semmes
Haze, 1994
Crushed rayon velvet

Fashion as the abstract expressionist sublime: the second skin of clothing flattened and smeared into a field of shimmering colour.

below right
Beverly Semmes created in collaboration with The Fabric Workshop and Museum, Philadelphia, *Watching Her Feat*, 2000
Nylon, stuffing (installation view with guard in matching dress)

Fabric is used for formal sculptural effects – shape, texture, dimension, colour – then compromised by its equivalence with the 'ordinary' body clad in the same material.

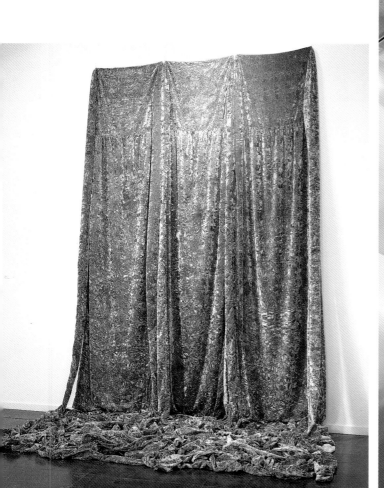

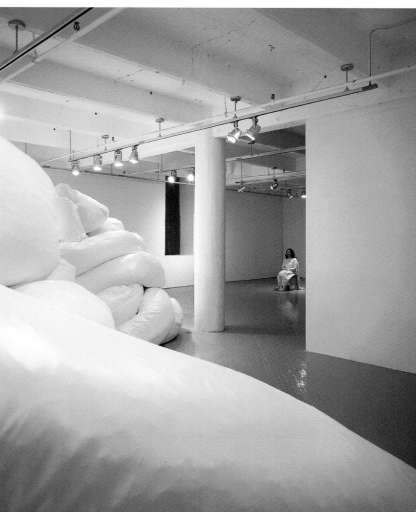

At first sight Beverly Semmes's installations of dresses, flattened against the gallery wall, hung high, their fabric trailing and pooling on the floor, can be understood as allusions to an absent body. Some body! What is evoked in pieces that may fall ten or fifteen feet is a body on such an improbable scale that we might read through its dimensions into a new domain – that of doubt. What bodies might inhabit these massively oversized garments? Semmes's clothes are larger than life and so come to assume lives of their own. They command attention to such a degree that, overwhelming the space which should structure and condition them, they initiate their own narratives. These stories may take their lead from the imagined body, in scenarios where the fabric, enlivened, comes to play a separate role, or, increasingly in Semmes's recent work, they may be based upon a contest, a formal engagement between volumes of fabric (which are also volumes of colour) and an almost encompassing space. To begin with there were bodies – the models in Semmes's photographic works of the late 1980s and early '90s who drifted through gardens and constructed landscapes in exotic, oversized hats and coats, becoming part of the environment through the agency of the clothing.

The use of fabric as story in itself is exemplified by the 1996 installation *Big Silver*, a vast dress in crushed silver lamé, raised and lowered against the gallery wall by motor-driven pulleys. Commissioned by the Smith College Museum of Art, this work was made in the wake of a collaboration between Semmes and the Mathilde Monnier dance company in France. In the summer of 1995 the artist made three sculptures inspired by movement in space. One of these was a long orange gown hung at the back of the stage, its fabric trailing towards the audience across the dance floor. Linda Muelhig noted that, 'As the dancers interacted with the dress, portions of the skirt were designed to detach and come away and, in a sense, to become part of the dance.'[1] Muelhig interprets *Big Silver* as a revival and transformation of Semmes's original intentions for the other two sculptures made for the Monnier company. Here the work becomes 'the active agent and locus of performance. Separated from the actual content of the stage, *Big Silver* can be seen to refer to the dance by enacting the repetitive regimen of the ballet barre in perpetual, deep pliés from floor to ceiling.'[2] There is a playful linguistic convergence in the plications of the rising and falling fabric and the exercises of the dancer which the cloth mimics. Other works, such as the massively proportioned *Red Dress*, 1992, with its 45-foot-long train flooding fabric across the gallery, are not only similarly spectacular in both colour and scale, but similarly solicitous of narratives to make themselves intelligible. However, as Margo Crutchfield observes, there may be a degree to which the work is 'comical, even ludicrous, with its grandiose posturing, as if pretending to be something it is not'.[3]

It is perhaps the paradoxes inherent in this Brobdignagian escalation that have guided Semmes towards an increased abstraction of material forms and a less pronounced emphasis upon the overtly corporeal. If Semmes's earlier works had appealed to an exaggerated (absent or absenting) body as armature, in much the same manner as Judith Shea – working on a human scale but away from the unstable materials of fashion into the permanence of the monument – the tendency towards formal emphases can be understood as abstracting *into* the very stuff of fashion. The questionable utility of garments on such a scale, with such internal structures, begs another question – that of form versus function. So it is that a work such as *Haze*, 1994, invokes a Rothko-like sublime. Just as Rothko spoke of his flat-field paintings as 'skins hung on the wall', so Semmes pushes the object – the second 'skin' of clothes – beyond its recognizable limits. *Haze* is still strangely pellicular, but barely recognizable as three conjoined dresses, their distended arms just breaking from a flattened, vertical plane to fall in a horizontal rectangle of compressed material. The flat field of shimmering colour is not, of course, manifold veils of translucent paint: Semmes conjures a similar abstraction from crushed rayon velvet, with a pattern... Nature from culture indeed!

Semmes's exhibition at Lesley Tonkonow Gallery in spring 2001 further emphasized the degree to which her employment of fashion's materials had shifted from concern with their representational, narrative possibilities towards more formal interests. *Watching Her Feat*, 2000, consisted of a large coil of luminescent yellow nylon, filled with styrofoam pellets, and occupying the main part of the gallery space. It was as if the pooled, crumpled trains of earlier dresses had become detached —·as in Semmes's piece for Monnier – and formed the sole object of attention. As if to redress the balance, Semmes insisted that the gallery staff wear matching outfits, of normal scale, throughout the exhibition. Where previously the artwork had spoken of the body in its absence, through scale, shape and colour, here there was a separation of form and function, on one hand returning utilitarian value to clothing, on the other emphasizing its properties of colour, texture and shape through abstraction.

If Beverly Semmes has, over the last decade, increasingly privileged form over function – partly by representing function as improbable – Karen Kimmel, over much the same period, has used the form of fashion to interrogate, and ironically mimic, social function. Making the audience smile, or even laugh, is an essential component of Kimmel's work. In an interview she commented, 'My art is meant to be humorous. When people look at one of my installations and say, "That's kind of silly," I say, "Exactly!" I don't expect to explain my work to someone and have them say, "Hmmm. Interesting. Profound." I expect them to laugh, smile and say, "How did you come up with that stupid idea?"'[4]

Is Kimmel's work, then, nothing more than a mime of an essential frivolity which haunts fashion (a mime which in the last two years has extended into fashion itself through her partnership in the exclusive Los Angeles clothing store K-Bond)? Kimmel's statement is itself permeated by a self-deprecating irony that extends the 'stupidity' of her work. Any accomplished writer of fiction will admit that often the most serious commentary can only be freighted into a text under the guise of comedy. Kimmel, too, is acutely aware of the overbearing profundity which can be escaped, and the subversive seriousness which can be communicated, through playing 'dumb', through making us smile at 'stupid' ideas. A stock more of literature, such strategies remain unusual in contemporary art. Despite the alleged frivolousness and parodic tendencies of postmodern culture, art remains a serious, unfunny practice, its very earnestness deterring public engagement. Kimmel is one of those rare living artists – with John Currin, perhaps, or Paul McCarthy – who can efface a serious critical imagination behind the mask of dumb humour. We laugh at the performance, and only later, slowly, does it dawn on us that the over-emphatic attention to detail, the exaggeration to the point of ridicule which amused us, carries with it the burden that these details are components of our quotidian lives to which we readily surrender.

Karen Kimmel
[open], 2001
Performers with silk pyjama sets,
silk pillowcases, silk eyemasks
with embroidery, straw slippers

The 'stupid' idea that through
a contextual irony draws our attention
to the social conditions of production
and the organization of social space,
[open] is a crazy simulacrum of
fashion's manufacture.

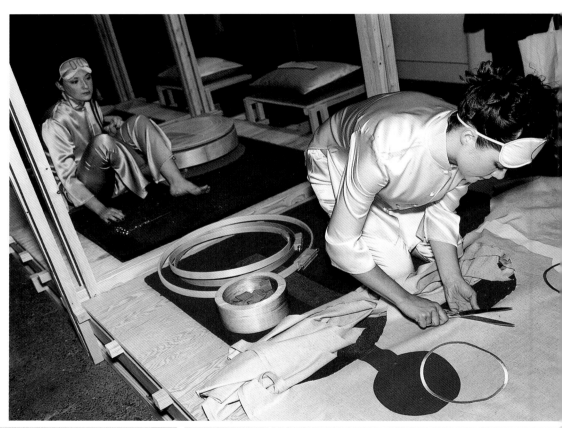

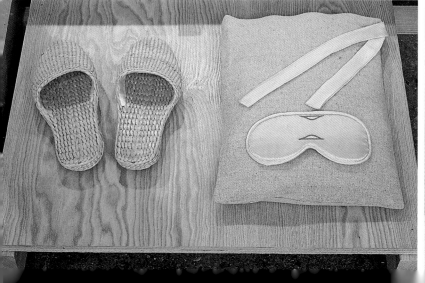

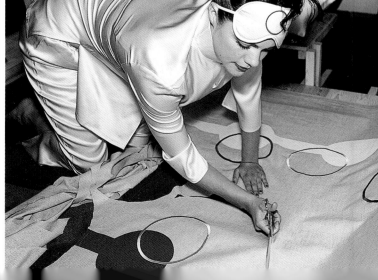

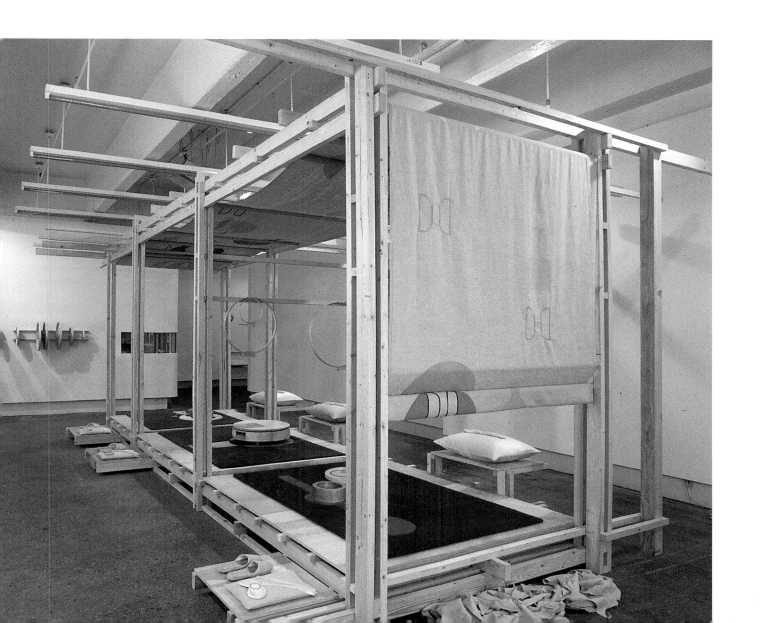

Kimmel's performances dwell upon the coding of the social domain by clothing, by the ways in which we contour ourselves to perform tasks through particular forms of fashion. Perhaps one of the surprises of her career is that she hasn't yet initiated an in-flight performance with air hostesses – but maybe that would be too obvious, an area where the forms of social costuming already tread a fine line between functionality and self-parody. In the late 1990s, however, Kimmel's performances did have that seductive, ephemeral quality of service that in-flight attendants uniquely offer. The provocation of temporary desire was fundamental to pieces such as *Savor* and *Quench*, both performed in 1997. These events worked much like product promotional exercises in public spaces: there was the free product – cold lemon-water in *Quench*, ice cream (vanilla or chocolate) in *Savor*; there were attractive attendants, strangely attired so that they were immediately noticeable; there were contexts of need. These performances were staged at exhibition openings – crowded, hot and intense social spaces where people need a drink, or, to distance themselves from both art and audience, the ice cream and tranquillity of the separate seating area that *Savor* provided. Central to these performances was a recognition by their audiences of being participants – rather than passive spectators – in a somewhat absurd event, coupled with an awareness that this participation necessitated their conformity, through desire, to the social situation that Kimmel had created. As Stuart Horodner noted of *Savor*, 'These outfits, chairs and pops [ice creams] ... were loaded accommodations that forced viewers to participate in the space between their own free will and Kimmel's restrictive conditioning.'[5]

The territory that Horodner describes is as much the conceptual field of subjectivity as it is the social domain of performance and event. This, in large measure, is both Kimmel's play area, the space of parody, and her 'serious' point – that subjectivity is structured by its willing participation in the bizarre rituals of the social sphere. These are observances which, subjected to a contextualized irony, placed in the 'wrong' space, or hyperbolized just so much, suddenly appear as preposterous. *Guide*, 1997, took this fondness for hyperbole and use value into the more general, diffuse space of the city for the first time. The performance was used to highlight sites in New York's 'Downtown Arts Festival'. *Guide* was, however, what Horodner described as 'a curious mapping, where the sign may be more interesting than the destination'.[6] The work used twelve women wearing white sleeveless tops, long pink skirts and white running shoes, each wearing a device on her back that unfurled a twenty-foot yellow banner, bearing a pink and orange arrow, and linking one performer umbilically to another. This chain of actants ostensibly provided a useful service as it roamed the southern end of Manhattan, guiding interested spectators to festival venues, but, as Horodner observed, offering spectators enough spectacle in itself to deflect attention from those sites.

Until recently few of Kimmel's performances had been concerned with self-sufficient systems of social signs: most relied upon audience involvement. An early exception was *step up *37*, 1998, in which female protagonists in laboratory coats positioned hanging objects in the performance space and then traced their silhouettes on its enclosing walls. This concern with the production of representation, as an abstracted system, was further developed in *[open]*, staged at Sara Meltzer's New York gallery in spring 2001. *[open]* can be seen as a parodic re-staging of both fashion and art's productions within the coding of the factory system. The decorative objects which that system generates, and which the gallery sells, are products of alienated labour in an economy that figures the artist as entrepreneur. Given their shared interest in a blank ironization of their artistic strategies – a public face of 'dumb', oh-gee humour – there can be little surprise in Kimmel's enterprise being debt-financed, as it were, by Warhol.

Like *step up *37*, [open] contains a tracing of objects, a performance of representation, within and on its walls. Like *step up *37*, [open] relies upon performers to literalize the social action of subjective language: making traces is equivalenced by making decorative fabric shapes. Where, however, the earlier piece provides a critical model of the social field as constraining language laboratory, [open] is a more overt critique, and perhaps a celebration, of the production process of luxury goods – whether those of art or fashion. If we buy a work of art from a well-dressed gallerist in an expensive, well-appointed white cube, we do not assume its producer to have participated in the stylistic economy of the gallery. Indeed, such a participation might disappoint our romantic notions of the artist as paint-spattered genius in a remote and equally dishevelled studio, indifferent to the selling prices of the objects that he or she creates. Similarly, if we buy a luxury fashion object in Bond Street or on the Upper East Side, we do not assume its producers to have participated in the stylistic economy of the store: we might also acknowledge that their connection to its fiscal economy is often marginal. We do not expect the producers of luxury goods to themselves be adorned in items of luxury, nor to use golden scissors – though this might be a utopian ideal of luxury. The women who work in the ateliers of the fashion industry are rarely as strikingly beautiful as the models Kimmel paid to be her workers. By dressing models in this way and by selling the products of their alienated labour as art objects, Kimmel created a crazily warped simulacrum of fashion's manufacture to emphasize the difference between what the object permits us to imagine, through consumption, and the actuality of social conditions of production, whether in art or fashion. These are idealized, functional systems which, through the very absurdity of that ideal and the very uselessness of their utilitarianism, draw attention to the character of the more quotidian systems in which we are enmeshed ●

[open] used three attractive models as 'workers', dressed in silk pyjamas, with matching sleep masks worn on the forehead as if they were industrial glasses or welding goggles. The 'overalls' of each worker were colour-coded according to their separate tasks in the division of labour: pink for 'The Chooser', pale green for 'The Stretcher' and taupe for 'The Appraiser'. Each role corresponded to a stage in the production of objects within an open wooden structure, carpeted, and with a spill of fine-grained, silk-screened and embroidered canvas, falling from ceiling to 'factory' floor. 'The Chooser' marked, measured and cut circles from the decorated fabric. These were passed to 'The Stretcher', who aligned the fabric on an embroidery hoop, stretched it taut and removed excess material with a pair of golden scissors. 'The Appraiser' – an equivalent perhaps of a quality controller – then checked the finished object, attached a price tag and hung the work onto a mount already fixed on the gallery wall.

8

DRESSING UP
DRESSING DOWN

SALES LESSON:
CLOTHING PACKAGES
INDIVIDUALS TO
ACHIEVE SUCCESS

Antony McCall and Andrew Tyndall
Argument, 1978

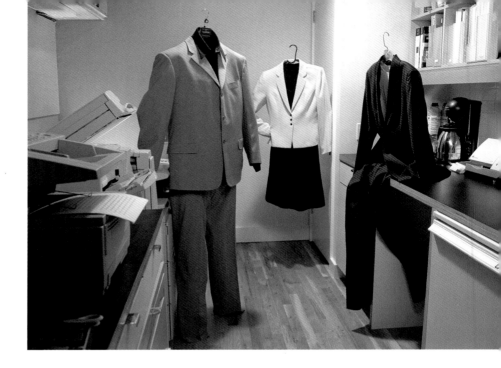

right
Maureen Connor
Copy Room, 2002
Digital print

opposite left
Maureen Connor
Conference Room, 2002
Digital print

opposite centre
Maureen Connor
Flying Clothes 2, 2002
Digital print

opposite below
Maureen Connor
Tired, 2002
Digital print

As long as your uniform conforms, who cares whether the body shows up? Just remember that anyone can fill your shoes, so long as the shoes fit in. In a variety of workplace situations, Connor depicts the clothes necessary to dress for success. Anyone can fit these uniforms; anyone can meet the corporate clothing requirement on dressing casually without expressing individuality. What really matters is obedience to regulation; the willingness to look the part rather than to be oneself. So there is no need for a self in these pictures. Clothes make the employee.

opposite far right above
Maureen Connor
From *Dress Down Friday*, 2002
Digital print

'The past is a foreign country. They do things differently there.' Or perhaps not. Connor's chart (above) adapts the regulations issued by sixteenth-century British monarchs (below) to govern who wore what, and where, to the strictures of contemporary corporate codes, and reveals that less has changed than you might imagine.

In the press of the crowd in the financial district of the City of London on a weekday morning you rapidly become accustomed to the recurrence of a few basic costumes: the secretary in prim chain-store suit and coat, and running shoes (heels, near impossible to walk in with safety on the capital's fractured pavements, are saved for the office portals); the senior executive in heavily pinstriped suit, its wool quality index-linked to salary and share options, complemented by a striped, double-cuffed shirt, a tie signifying membership of an established institution such as a gentleman's club, or else of the old, private school. More junior, still aspirant traders and managers adhere to this code, and play with it; the suit may be plain, more nuanced in its cut and detail – perhaps an extravagant five buttons on the cuffs; the shirt and tie, too, will be more subtly experimental, adhering to the conventions of corporate life and social status whilst announcing difference. Still further down the hierarchy, and perhaps accompanying a shift of functions from actuarial to clerical, you notice – just – the men in grey, the utilitarian suit and shirt and tie and shoes, where benchmark sameness is compromised only by the wearing of socks printed perhaps with a teddy bear motif. Occasionally you might observe, reflected in a shop window, the idiosyncratic, self-reflexive figure of the art historian, trying to make sense of this world and subverting its vestimentary orders with the inverted seams and unfinished

buttonholes of a Demeulemeester suit and scarlet boots from Alessandro dell'Acqua. You could, on a grander or lesser scale, repeat the same walk in most other Western cities, around Wall Street or the Paris *bourse*. There would be national distinctions. There might be, especially in New York, the regulated observance of a corporate dress code rather than the equally constrained but tacit conformance of London's Square Mile. But everywhere you would observe a close adherence to a set of expectations of what a man or woman, doing a particular job, is meant to look like, in order to appear responsible and professional, in order to be successful.

Walk around these areas on one particular working day, however, and you will observe a radical change. Those senior managers will still be there in Brooks Brothers or Gieves & Hawkes, but the lower orders will have been transformed. It is 'Dress Down Friday' – 'Casual Friday' if you are on Wall Street – an informal and still evolving development in business dress codes, which allows staff at the end of the working week the opportunity to appear at the office in more informal, more personal clothing. What you'll also notice, however, is how much the same everyone looks; how the gradations, restrictions and distinctions of the suit are transferred onto casualwear. All of the men are wearing chinos, sports shirts and casual jackets. Ripped jeans, leather jackets and motorcycle

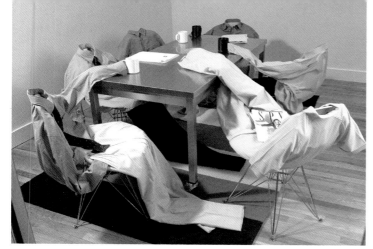

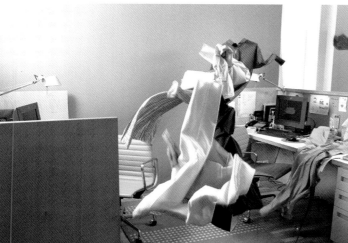

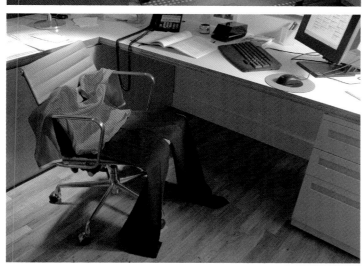

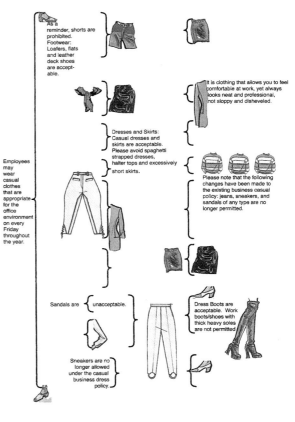

As a reminder, shorts are prohibited. Footwear: Loafers, flats and leather deck shoes are acceptable.

It is clothing that allows you to feel comfortable at work, yet always looks neat and professional, not sloppy and disheveled.

Dresses and Skirts: Casual dresses and skirts are acceptable. Please avoid spaghetti strapped dresses, halter tops and excessively short skirts.

Please note that the following changes have been made to the existing business casual policy: jeans, sneakers, and sandals of any type are no longer permitted.

Employees may wear casual clothes that are appropriate for the office environment on every Friday throughout the year.

Sandals are unacceptable.

Dress Boots are acceptable. Work boots/shoes with thick heavy soles are not permitted

Sneakers are no longer allowed under the casual business dress policy.

MEN'S APPAREL

NONE SHALL WEAR			
Cloth of gold, Silver tissue, Silk of purple colour		Except	Earls and above that rank, and Knights of the Garter in their purple mantles.
Cloth of gold or silver, tinselled satin, silk or cloth mixed or embroidered with gold or silver. Foreign woollen cloth		Except	Barons and above that rank. Knights of Garter, and Privy Councillors.
Any lace of gold or silver, mixed with gold and silver, or with gold or silver and silk.		Except	Barons' sons and all above that rank. Gentlemen attending upon the Queen in house or chamber. Those who have been employed in embassies. Those with net income of 500 marks per year for life. Knights (as regards daggers, spurs, etc.); Captains.
Spurs, swords, rapiers, daggers, buckles or studs of girdles, etc.	Gilt or damasked with gold or silver silvered		
Velvet in	Gowns Cloaks Coats and upper garments	Except	Knights and all above that rank; their heirs apparent; those with net income of £200, and all excepted in preceding article.
Embroidered with silk Netherstocks of silk			
Velvet in	Jerkins Hose Doublets		
Satin Damask Taffeta Grograin	in	Gowns Cloaks Coats, etc.	Except	Knights' eldest sons, and all above that rank. Those with net income of £100. Those excepted above.
Velvet Gilding Silvering, etc. Studs Buckles, or other garniture, gilt, silvered, etc.	in	Saddles Bridles Stirrups, and all furniture of horse	Except	Barons' sons and all above that rank; Knights; Men with incomes of 500 marks etc. as above.

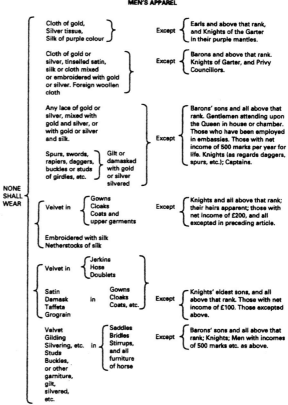

boots are not common sights, any day of the week, except on couriers and art historians. As Maureen Connor puts it, 'Although designed to allow more freedom and comfort, the advent of "Dress Down Friday" has created, paradoxically (as is almost always the case with fashion), the need for an entirely new set of sartorial rules and codes.'[1]

Connor's most recent project, the installation *Dress Down Friday*, explores the immediate condition of these codes and how the subversion of formality that the legitimized dissent of 'dressing down' seemed to promise has itself become a formal exercise in which the sartorial signification of status and aspiration is at least as important as that articulated by conventional businesswear. Connor's work also highlights the strange historical continuities presented by the regulation of employees' appearance by corporations, whether through written codes devised by 'human resources' departments or the unspoken tenets of peer pressure.

What is now manifested as control at the corporate level was once a pressing responsibility for the emergent state. From late medieval times well into the early modern era, the appearance of individuals was, to a varying degree, regulated through national and local sumptuary laws. This control of individual appearance reflected two principal anxieties, both connected to the rapid accumulation of wealth in emerging capitalist economies. Firstly there was a fear of opulent display amongst women in cultures which largely associated demure appearance with chastity, and secondly there was a concern with 'passing', whereby newly enriched merchants and tradesmen might appear as aristocrats because of their costume and newly-learned social graces. (Albrecht Dürer was making such a move in his first painted self-portrait, presented in pre-nuptial negotiations – itself an aristocratic practice – depicting himself in the guise of an eligible young courtier. Dürer came from a family of artisans – goldsmiths – and at the time was only an itinerant painter. Art, like fashion, lied about its subject.) Such legislation was, unlike earlier regulation, too late to control the phenomenon. As Connor remarks, 'Renaissance sumptuary laws contrast with other institutional dress codes in that they were enacted after the fact – as an attempt to control hierarchies that were already destabilized.'[2]

State legislation and contemporary corporate policy both seek to regulate fashion's capacity to make statements about its wearer. In the former case there is an interest in maintaining the social order by insisting upon modesty, or presentability, and truth. In our time, presentability surfaces once again as a fundamental issue: corporations are not necessarily policing social hierarchies, but are, rather, concerned with maintaining an appropriate image for their clients. This image is achieved at the cost of constraint upon the individual. Maureen Connor's project suggests that even as 'Dress Down Friday' constitutes a moment of carnival – a temporary, licensed dissent from the norms of business dress codes – the phenomenon is a similar attempt to contain the cultural displacements of contemporary economic life as they are reflected, however darkly, in fashion.

'Dress Down Friday' has rapidly produced its own complex of acceptable appearances and sartorial niceties. In the last five years 'Dressing Down' has spawned a multitude of image consultants, fashion shows targeted at the managerial classes, and 'how to' publications which parallel the explosion in Renaissance Italy of conduct manuals, advising on everything from table manners to appropriate dress,[3] and a new emphasis on exterior appearance as a reflection of both social status and individual identity. Whereas in the 1980s men and women power-dressed for success, by the late '90s mainstream publishers were promoting titles such as *Dress Casually for Success for Men*.[4] Maureen Connor's striking artistic anthropology of power and aesthetics in the contemporary workplace is also an archaeology that reveals profound continuities between past and present.

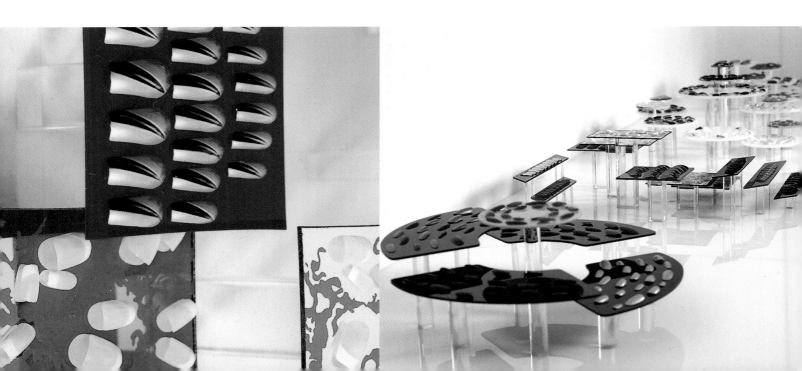

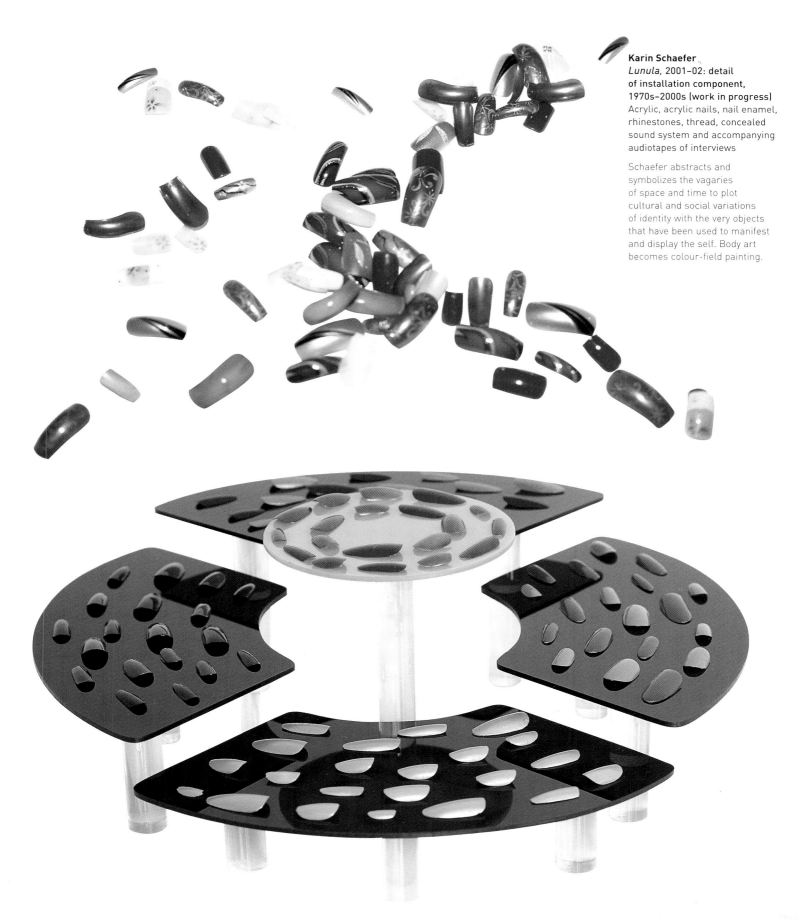

Karin Schaefer
Lunula, 2001–02: detail
of installation component,
1970s–2000s (work in progress)
Acrylic, acrylic nails, nail enamel,
rhinestones, thread, concealed
sound system and accompanying
audiotapes of interviews

Schaefer abstracts and
symbolizes the vagaries
of space and time to plot
cultural and social variations
of identity with the very objects
that have been used to manifest
and display the self. Body art
becomes colour-field painting.

Karin Schaefer's installation *Lunula* explores one detail of personal appearance: the fingernail. In the last twenty years, especially in the United States, a culture of decoration has developed upon this small and easily overlooked body site. The nails are richly embellished, painted with 'polish' in elaborate formal and expressive patterns, and also 'sculpted' with rhinestones, jewelry and acrylic. At the same time as these images reflect the wearer's mood and personality, the changes that have occurred in the palette of available colours and styles of decoration graph fluctuations in the aesthetic values of popular culture. *Lunula* is a map – itself highly decorative – that plots those cultural and social variations through the objects of nail art. Schaefer takes the map, itself a symbolization of space and time, and abstracts it a stage further. For Schaefer, this project is both 'an anthropological investigation and immersion into the beauty industry's reflection and influence on our state of being' and 'a playful exploration of color and form' through the iconography of nail decoration.[5]

Schaefer organizes hundreds of painted nails in chronological order and particular arrangements to reflect the shifting patterns of taste and fashion. Colours and styles range from the punk and disco glamour of the mid-1970s, through the reds and blacks and accompanying decorative extravagance of the '80s, and the rich dark colours of the early '90s, to the 'techno'-influenced colours such as cement and taupe of the late '90s, and contemporary hues. Schaefer's art of cultural history highlights an ongoing exchange between sub-cultural expression and the trends set by mainstream manufacturers. As the artist points out, 'From the seventies onward punk and the counter culture introduced blues and other colors that had traditionally not been associated with nail polish. By the late nineties Chanel – the arbiter of high fashion in nail decoration – had a blue as their top selling color.'[6]

Nail decoration reflects a particular investment in the desire for individual appearance; a desire that, as Schaefer illustrates, is often structured by class, age and ethnicity. The colours and patterns that are chosen are the consequences of an extensive and often time-consuming process to find the perfect style for a specific event, or a more generalized image that the individual wants to project to the world. An audio loop around the display cases of *Lunula* carries the voices of women from diverse backgrounds and of all ages, as well as those of the manicurists who carry out this detailed and exacting art as work. Clients and practitioners talk about the investments they make in the iconography of this decorative form, and the degree to which the polished nail reflects their understanding of their true identities.

Charles LeDray's meticulous reproductions of clothes, hung from equally carefully crafted hangers, court the risk of any miniature: in the reduction of use value the spectator's response is to acclaim the craft of its negation, the attention to detail in the diminution of the real. This courting is perhaps deliberate – a danger that the form of the work embodies and subverts. LeDray's work – and it is important to insist on it as 'work' – is all his own. Taught to sew at the age of four by his mother, the artist subsequently trained himself to fashion other materials into tiny replicas of real, crafted or industrially manufactured objects. Such skill may provoke sentimentality as its consequence. In condensing the world, miniaturization literalizes the processes of metonymy, making 'digestible' those effects and objects that are too large for us to incorporate, but with which we nonetheless identify, which we want to be part of ourselves. Experience is understood and accommodated either through its fragments, which may seem to us enlarged (the process of synecdoche) or through a form of metaphor in which the whole is condensed into the part (the metonym). LeDray's work can be understood

as metonymical in its condensation and as explanatory of metonymy in its explicitly miniaturized rendering of the world. And sentimentality – as sympathy with an otherness in which we see something of ourselves, without ever really comprehending its true nature – is both effect and mechanism of this process of identification.

In replicating clothes, however, LeDray is perhaps more interested in symbolizing their diverse, contestatory messages than he is with the technical and formal questions of scaling down the real to manageable proportions. These are clearly not the clothes of the doll's house. Rather LeDray resorts to the miniature in part as critique of the trivialization and condensation of experience that the replication of history also effects. The application of 'pointless' labour to 'trivial' detail, the absorption of play and work, and of play into work, emphasizes the degree to which fashion shuttles between fantasy and reality. As LeDray comments of his creations, they are 'fully realized works, but not fully real'.[7] In re-fashioning fashion, LeDray undertakes a challenge both to the meaning of clothes and to the meaning of metonymy. Complementing the ambivalent status of the miniature, there is sometimes a deliberate aggression against it as 'beautiful, useless object' which is simultaneously a violence against the larger meanings that the miniature might encode.

This is perhaps most obvious in *Untitled*, 1995. The outfit is that of a 'gentleman': to an Englishman it might embody tradition, conservatism, a longstanding relationship to the land and a position of authority within it. The costume might also signify a particular relationship to, and propagation of, knowledge that is itself profoundly traditional, rooted more in the observance of ritual than in critical enquiry. There are many Oxbridge academics who today would still unquestioningly wear clothes such as these, almost as a uniform. Perhaps all that LeDray omits is a perfectly crafted pair of punched brown leather brogues. For an American

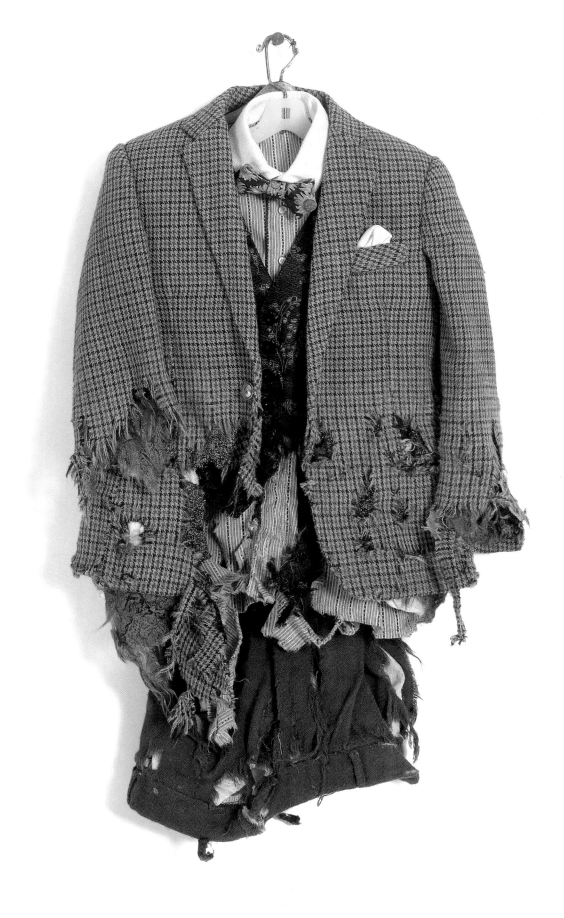

Charles LeDray
Untitled, 1995
Fabric, thread, plastic, paint, wood, wire, gold-plated brass buttons

A deliberate condensation; a deliberate violence. LeDray examines the processes by which we understand and accommodate experience, then he disrupts them. One outfit epitomizes and undermines all that Ralph Lauren spent more than a decade and a slew of dollars to convey.

119

Alex Bag
Untitled (The Fashion Show),
from *Untitled (Spring '94)*, 1994
Video still

Alex Bag
Untitled (White Radio Girls),
from *Untitled (Spring '94)*, 1994
Video still

A manic, joyous ride through
a mass culture peopled by
fashion mavens, obsessive and
disinterested 'retail assistants'
and shopaholics; a world in
which everyone is a wannabe,
and where everyone wears
Wannabes. Bag topples every
carefully constructed pose into
an expository burlesque, but only
because she loves her subjects;
only because she, too, sees this
culture from the inside.

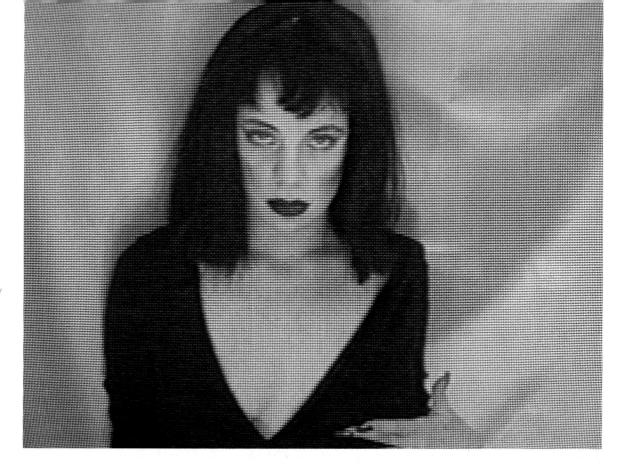

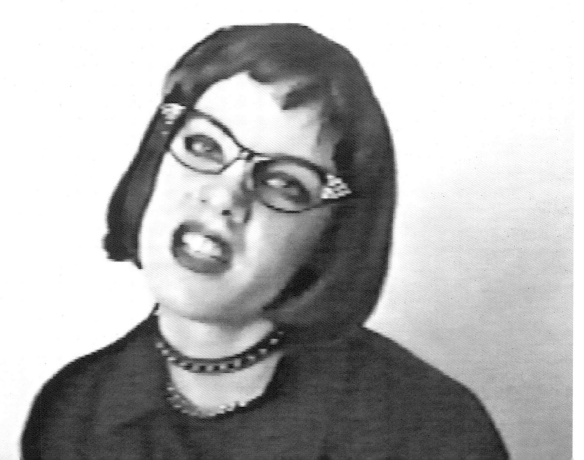

such an outfit provokes additional and historically differential readings: it announces itself as the garb of New England conservatism, of the preppy, and of a relationship to English tradition through a kind of aristocratic lineage. LeDray successfully condenses in one scaled-down outfit all that Ralph Lauren spent most of the 1980s and early '90s trying to convey in several collections, a slew of international stores and millions of dollars in advertising.

LeDray's use of sandpaper to fray and tear the detailed perfection he created is not only a mechanism that deters sentimental response. This meditated abrasion is a reaction to what the clothes stand for, their social values and their repression of other, more polymorphous, identities. Where Maureen Connor's recent project dwells upon the historical perpetuation of social construction through fashion and its regulation, LeDray's assault upon the replication of costume might be understood as a blow for individual, artistic liberation. The extraordinary 'self-portrait' *Charles*, 1995 – a miniature name-tagged janitor's uniform from which are suspended even smaller items of clothing, including dressing gowns, shirts, cardigans and brassières – suggests not only the liberating proliferation and diversification of LeDray's production as artist, but also the potential proliferation and diversification of identity that the buttoned-up conservatism of *Untitled*, 1995, would constrain.

Where Maureen Connor and Karin Schaefer chart the historical and spatial contours of fashion's effects, and Charles LeDray both condenses and violates them, Alex Bag is perhaps more intimate with the subjects of

her art. Bag climbs aboard and goes along for a ride through contemporary mass culture. The artist's videos are the confessions to camera of the (un)thinking life of fictional but oh so frighteningly real personae. In her engagement with the subjects of consumer culture, Bag recycles Pop art's delight in the mass object, via MTV and the Shopping Channel, into an art that is vibrant, alluring and alarming.

In *Spring '94*, Bag dissolves herself into the tell-all fervour of a fashion maven in full lather over the delights of Azzedine Alaïa's latest designs. In raven-black wig, haunted (and haunting) make-up, and with nails like extended talons, Bag exaggerates the pose of fashion TV's presenters into burlesque – after all, Cindy Crawford was never like this. And yet Bag's act is not simply painful parody; it is also painfully truthful in its exposé of obsession with ephemera. There are people out there, like this, living in the media world, as producers of desire, and living for it, as consumers. Furthermore, Bag suggests, if only by the degrees of sympathy necessary for her to occupy these characters, neither they nor the subjects of their passions are wholly abhorrent. In order to critique you have first to love, or at least be moved by the subject of your criticism. If Bag's mimicry was simple negation of consumer and object, it would not be so effective. There is a duplicitous delight in and repulsion by the exciting objects of seduction that constitute fashion.

Fall '95, Bag's follow-up work, not only delved further into the domains of mass culture, it began to explore the mindsets of its consumers as much as its promoters.

'Shopgirls' took the spectator inside the MTV world of a sales-girl who also plays in a rock band. This was a clever confection of artistic life-support (since most artists in whatever medium have at some point resorted to mediastine[8] roles, and wondered, immediately, if they would ever escape them), of the helpless longing for celebrity encouraged by contemporary mass media, and of the mid-decade convergence of popular music, fashion and art. By the early 1990s rock luminaries such as Kim Gordon of Sonic Youth were gracing fashion adverts and the occasional catwalk when touring commitments allowed. They were also going into the fashion business themselves (Gordon creating the X-Girl brand) or being seen in absolutely the right cutting-edge clothes (Courtney Love and Melissa auf der Maur of Hole both turning to the sculpted-on-the-body, performance-derived creations of Elisa Jimenez). To accentuate the point, *Fall '95*'s first showing was accompanied by footage culled from Bag's own collection of videos. This footage included Courtney Love herself – and Love was a great lookalike for Bag's shopgirl – Helmut Lang, Mary Quant advertisements and part of a film about the designer Stephen Sprouse.

Bag's construction of herself as other(s) depends upon a reduction of her medium – television – to an absurd and banal baseline, and then a return from bathetic parody, through a video bricolage, which far from romanticizing or disparaging its characters, deals in a sympathetic and horrified way with the self as a failed copy of the mediated ideal. Bag's personae are snapshots from inside, as much as they are films from outside, of the way we are now. They offer us – as art – cognitive maps of fashion's consumers ●

WHO WILL YOU BE TODAY?

9

GETTING DRESSED
IS NEVER
A SIMPLE MATTER

Catherine Liu

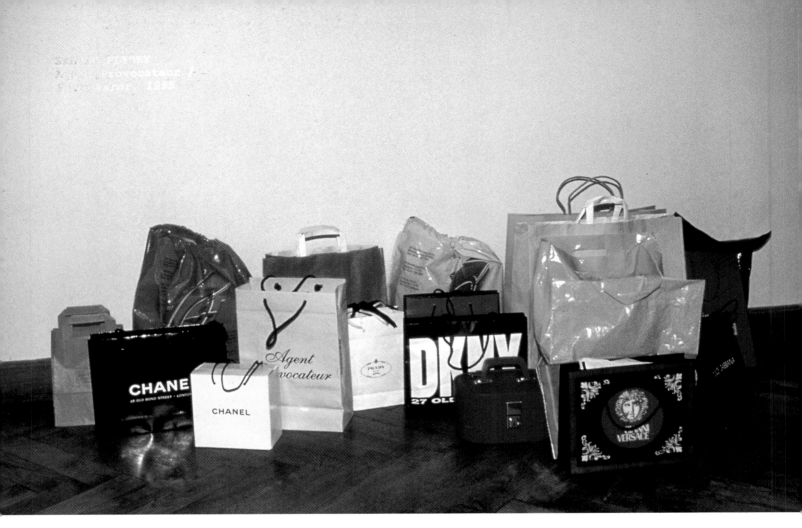

SYLVIE FLEURY
Agent Provocateur /
Pleasure Vapor, 1995

Sylvie Fleury
Agent Provocateur, 1995
Shopping bags and contents

'I shop therefore I am.' Fleury
satirizes the performance of
purchase, the enslavement to
the espadrille. Perhaps carrying
the bags says more about us than
the clothes inside. The designer
logo promises an identity that is
never quite achieved.

Sylvie Fleury
Moisturizing is the Answer, 1996
Neon sign

Endlessly repeated, the
advertising sign becomes a
religious mantra; the object
of a perfect faith in one's own
perfectibility. In repetition Fleury
gestures towards the growing
distance between the promises
of unfulfilled belief and the
possibilities of daily decrepitude.

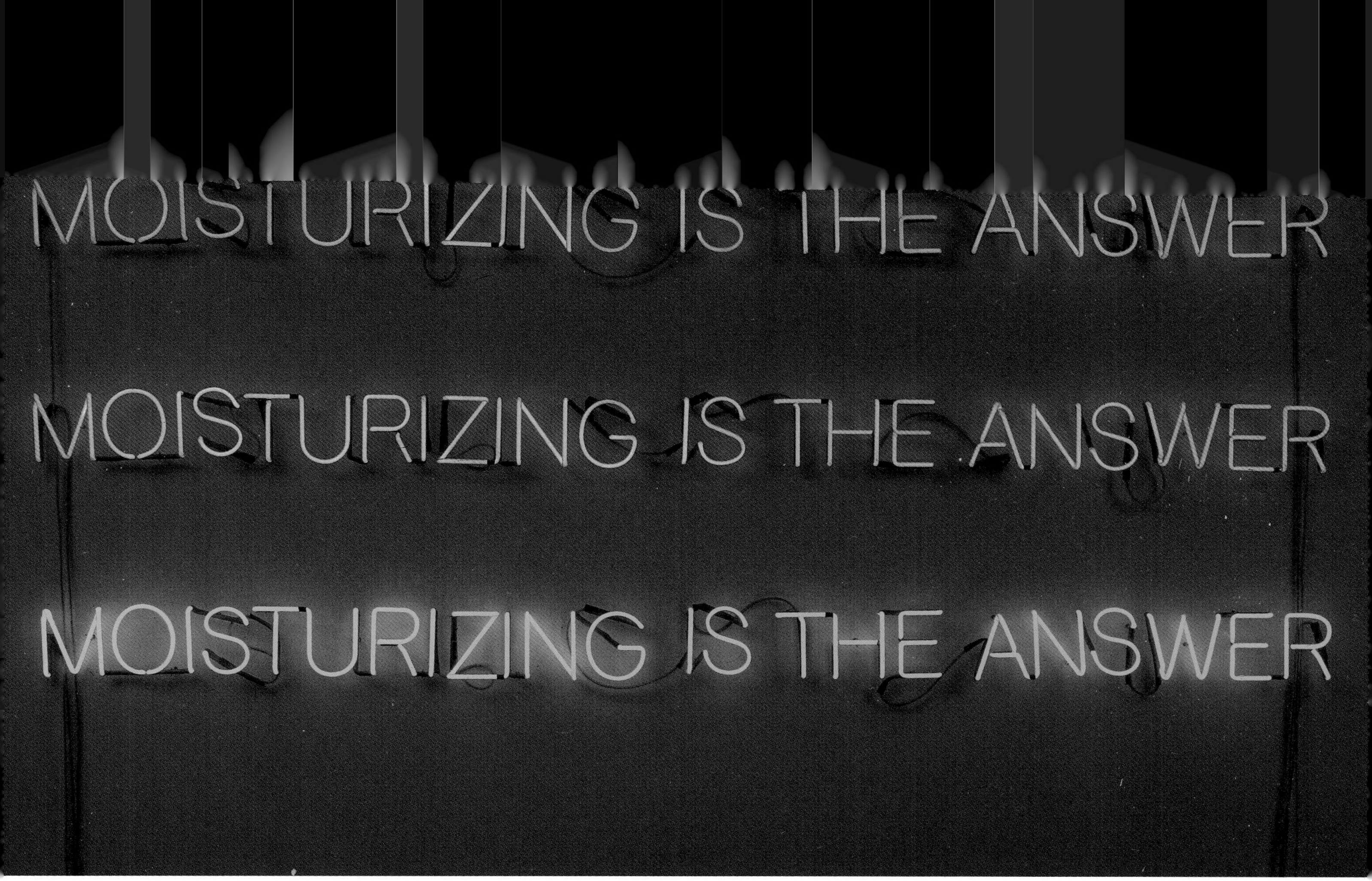

MOISTURIZING IS THE ANSWER

MOISTURIZING IS THE ANSWER

MOISTURIZING IS THE ANSWER

Identity *is* ready-to-wear. What might have been imagined as unique – a set of attributes that came with us, whether by nature, nurture, or some combination, and that we called our selves – is a condition that can be slipped from a hanger, lifted from a box, brought down from a shelf. And paid for with a credit card. The new identity of which clothes are tokens can be acquired in advance, much like Dürer with his betrothal portrait anticipating new class, new wealth, new status (see p. 116). Becoming 'yourself' is an investment – or, at least, given the plethora of style counsellors in New York and London, so you'd think.

When Sylvie Fleury, in her video *Twinkle*, 1992, endlessly tries on shoes, and we see only her feet prised into pair after pair after pair, what we are looking at is not simply a satire on the plethora of choices available in commodity culture, its wanton surfeit of product and possible identity, but a

meditation on the impossibility of making a correct choice, one that you control. You might be in your shoes, but simultaneously your shoes wear you. Fleury claims that no shopping trip is complete without the purchase of at least one pair of shoes. That, if we can afford the investment, is the alluring promise of the fashion object: a new identity every week, or at least with every pay cheque, if we want one. So, even if identity is what we wear, it is simultaneously disposable and contingent. Our clothes may tell no truths about us, other than to declare our own brittle whimsy. There may be no truth to tell. Buying, whether it is a dress or jewelry, promises to change your life, temporarily. As the advertisements for Patek Philippe watches put it, 'Who will you be in the next 24 hours?'

Advertisements for such personal transience are almost exclusively directed at women and depict female models. They suggest, if only

by their exclusion of the male, that there are different specificities of being: that femininity might involve being more 'naturally' ephemeral, constructed and performative than masculinity, where identity, like the body, is constrained by a narrower choice of clothing. Perhaps, such advertisements imply, women are the adventurous, mobile and imaginative performers of their selves against the rarely changing, settled backdrop of masculinity. If you are a man, the chances are that you'll be the same yesterday, today, tomorrow and so will your clothes – the last word against which the constantly mutable representations of feminine signification always stop.

The bags that Fleury assembles in installations such as *Agent Provocateur*, 1995, are bearers of unfulfilled promises. Those unopened packages of unworn clothes promise a new, transitory identity, just as soon as you open them and try the contents on. But those bags also represent a limit of meaning. The logo matters more than you do – if you can ever decide who 'you' are. Hugely glamorous, yet wholly disposable items, the carriers of Versace, Chanel, Prada and myriad others conspect consumption and spectacle. These tokens of the object are, to the untutored eye, more obvious a declaration of taste and wealth than the garments they contain. We know you buy Prada because the bag says so, even if what you are wearing is last season's Top Shop. What is inside the bag, as we bear it home, may never be seen. The container can confirm our difference, our glamour, to the rest of the world even when the contents cannot. So the carrier bag becomes a public display of possibility; the sign of a transformation of the body and identity which may be infinitely deferred, perhaps because the item is never worn, perhaps because it is only worn within, worn unseen. Hidden, the garment assumes a private meaning for each wearer – written in an introspective language – in a place where it cannot be interpreted and yet still demands interpretation. The signification of clothing may be simultaneously directed two ways – to private and public domains. Even as the heavily branded shopping bag, with its assertion of the company logo declares to the watching world that this new object is now

part of the bearer's identity, what is 'written' as being within the bag also signifies within. Such interiority may be literal: who sees us only in our underwear? Agent Provocateur is, after all, a designer label for garments worn close to the body, seen only by those with whom we are most intimate – our lovers, our doctors, our stalkers. The exchange of meaning provoked by the fashion object is brief, and supplements another exchange which the wearing, and perhaps the purchase, anticipates. Provocation is itself provoked. The bag, however, is another provocation altogether: a declaration of wealth and taste, to be sure, but also a public announcement of the future act, a broadcast of forthcoming intimacy.

Fleury's installations code these messages – their economies of sexuality, identity and wealth – and register them in public space – or rather in the gallery, a space perhaps more private than the street where they would otherwise be borne. But the external signification that the bags offer is not identical with the signification they contain; a signification whose possibility they disclose but never actually reveal. The meaning of clothes, both public and private, is maintained in part as a secret. Fleury's assemblages, which at a cursory glance seem to ironize spectacle and consumption,

are also sophisticated plays with the ambivalence of fashion's language – its encryption of our identities, the meanings we project onto our bodies through its effects. This play becomes more flagrant if we notice that the bags often remain sealed. Fleury promises us that the objects are still within, still perfect, still waiting to be worn. However, without opening the bags and destroying the perfection of the work, we can never know the truth of her assertion. That truth is 'saved', interiorized, for Fleury, who flippantly remarks that she always buys the garments in her size so that, if a 'work' does not sell, she can use its contents as clothes. Completed, however, the work of art constitutes the continual deferral of fashion's meaning. The bag becomes a burial chamber for clothes that will never be worn, identity that will never be realized. Here Fleury simultaneously denies and emphasizes the use value of fashion – which is not a utilitarian value as clothing, but rather a supplement to the body that initiates and apprehends a re-statement of identity.

If *Twinkle* represents an eternal deferral of choosing an identity, *Agent Provocateur* and similar projects presume that you have got over that particular hurdle. Instead they constitute an indefinite deferral of wearing what you have chosen – you never become what you think you want to be. Instead, by postponing that potential, Fleury points to its effect as meaning for the self through the absence of clothes. Fashion's function as sign of the self is thus displaced into another register. Displayed in a gallery, the shopping bag is a full yet empty statement; a commentary on fashion as statement rather than a fashion statement.

The deferral of fashion's bodily supplements and transformations transfers them, still as objects of consumption, into another domain – that of art. Here consumption is, of course, another statement about the self and the construction of identity through acquisition, and a particular display of economies that are both fiscal and subjective. The use value of the sign is sustained, but its new field of recognition necessitates a changed function: in a critique of the transaction within the art market we might see it now as a fiscal multiplier rather than the subjective increment that the garment represents. (To buy, as art, the clothes in bags that you will never wear, will cost you rather more than if you purchase them as wearable fashion.)

But this translation of the fashion object into art's field of meaning has a further effect.

If the artwork 'works', the garments remain inside their bags, useless and still enfolded in their tissue. Thus encrypted, they are forever perfect, their death infinitely demurred. These clothes will never wear out, get stained or torn; never acquire that sense of sameness with the world that sooner or later affects all new garments, no matter how beautiful, how glamorous, how expensive. Their perfection is guaranteed because they never enter the world. If identity is indeed 'ready-to-wear', then Fleury's installations provoke reflection on that identity and at the same time insist on its refusal. To begin is to acknowledge that there will be an ending. Never to open the crypt where these signs of life are buried is to presume infinitude because communication – decryption – never begins. If fashion is a continual turnover of novelty – novelty initiated by resuscitations of the past – these assemblages intervene in that economy by blocking the cycle – burying the object and refusing to begin the circuit of transformations that ends in death, first for fashion's garments and ultimately for the body.

Fleury's games with fashion's signs immure the ready-to-wear body behind the logos in which it has so enthusiastically invested. By contrast, Elisa Jimenez's dresses court

a borderline between the condition of art and the condition of fashion, so that the sculpted is worn and the worn sculpted. Everything depends on the body. There is nothing about Jimenez's work that is 'ready-to-wear', unless it is the form on which the dress is built. As New York fashion writer April Hughes puts it, 'Jimenez is all about handmade: from her tattoos, personally done by her best friend, to the perfect pair of sparkly jeans, she's the definitive manual labor aficionado.'[1]

Jimenez began her career as a performance artist, creating semi-fictional personae about her own body in a narrative construction she called 'The Hunger World'. That projection of identity involved certain fabrications – both the capacity to dissimulate and elaborate the self, and the need for costumes as rhetorical forms to articulate those deceptions and mythologies. Jimenez's self-designed dresses first became integral parts of her performances, then attained an objective status of their own. The formal handmade elements of the garments, their relations to, and significations of, the body, were recognized as 'sculptural'. Those same characteristics attracted individuals who also sought to fix the identifications attached to Jimenez's dresses in performative contexts. Their 'fix'

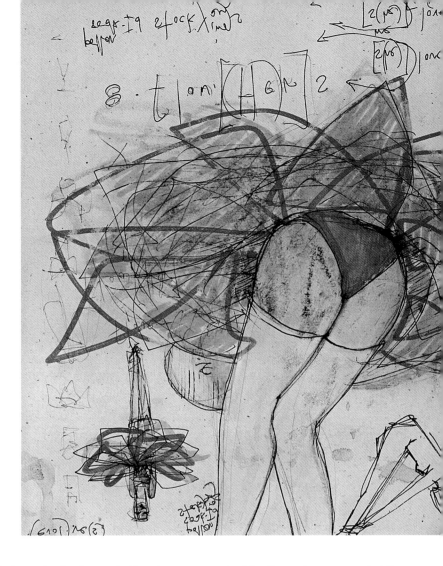

was the purchase: 'unfixed' was the significatory value of the garment, not only through its reconstitution in another environment, but also through a mutability embodied in its creation. This mutability is realized not only in the improvisatory process of construction on the body without pattern ('If something rips, it's how you deal with it,'[2] as Jimenez says), it is present in the adaptability of the garment, so that a halterneck dress folds successively into a wrap skirt or strapless tube, a one-shouldered gown and a high-necked column.

Jimenez's performances were not catwalk shows designed to display her 'products', although now as a maker of fashion, her catwalk shows *are* performance art. The caption for a *New York Times* picture of *Her Wild Horse Heart Matrix*, a 1999 performance in Williamsburg, describes the event as a 'fashion happening'. This is a neat conflation

of the design and collective production of clothes contingent on the performance into a tradition of post-war 'event art' in which any one performance might employ a variety of media and artists, contain no readily discernible narrative trajectory, and might – at least in the popular imagination – be suffused with a sense of the erotic and gradually spiral into chaos. The twenty or more performers of *Her Wild Horse Heart Matrix* were dressed in, amongst other garments, a purple and white heart dress, 'extremely slinky, low-cut down the back and high cut up the side of [the] legs',[3] marinated in red wine, whisky and sugar. Accompanying the charge of 'horse' performers around an old warehouse were a drummer – one of the few male participants – and an opera singer.

Whilst in certain aspects of content, mediation and location – using both marginal and novel venues – Jimenez's performances do reiterate

aspects of the Happening movement of the early 1960s, there are other elements, not least their emphasis on female corporeality and ritual, which place them firmly in a tradition of feminist art. Many of the more radical aspects of art associated with the women's movement in the decade following the mid-1970s rested upon a belief in the prehistoric figure of the Great Mother and concepts of matriarchal power, coupled with deeply romanticized notions of 'primitive' authenticity, proximity to nature and orgiastic rites as oppositions to patriarchal values. As Lucy Lippard put it in one of the works that promulgated this historically suspect notion of femininity as 'nature' in opposition to masculinity as 'culture', these associations and their realization in artworks were part of 'women artists' attempts to *restore* a forceful female image'.[4] In its emphasis upon a return to primal values and universal truths of existence, much of this discourse now reads

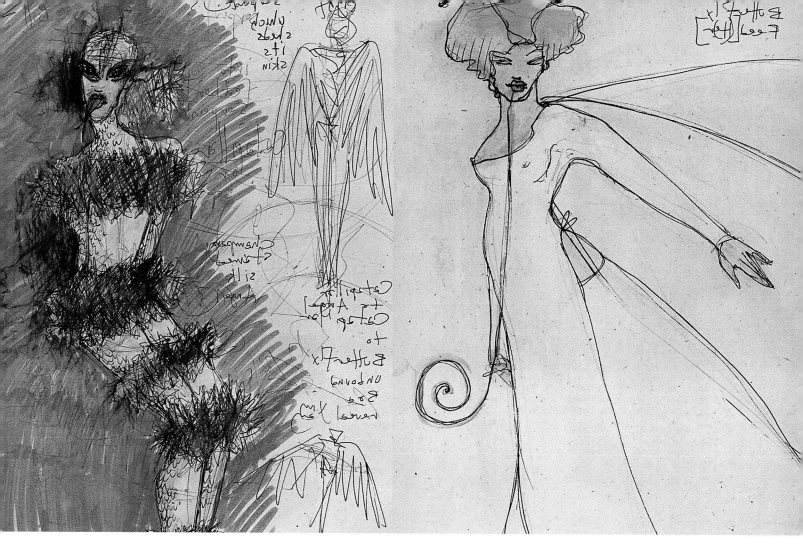

like the theoretical precepts of Abstract Expressionism rearticulated within feminist performance. Within both these recourses to the primitive and the essential, there is manifest a desire to arrest meaning, to reach a universal and transcendent signifier, whether the female body or a collective unconscious.

Jimenez's performances, including *Claiming the Sacred Harlot, In the Woods... Well-Come-Bliss-Dawn* and *Her Wild Horse Heart Matrix*, make public what were, in the 1970s, essentially private events in 'sacred' places, such as Jane Gilmor's oracular performances at Delphi. Furthermore, Jimenez locates ritual *within* culture: hers are events which work outwards into new social domains, not least through the dissemination of clothes in economies of exchange that are often not fiscal.[5] Women's art of the 1970s and '80s, where it attends to

Elisa Jimenez
Working drawings for performance, September 2001
Watercolour, pen and ink

Sketches for costumes to be worn in a mythical narrative which become, through the impact of performance, costumes to be worn by other performers, enacting other fantasies, in the real world.

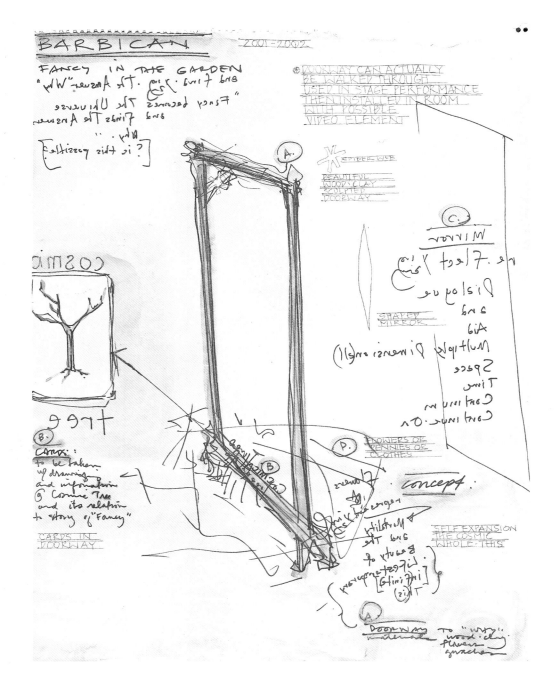

Some text in the drawing (partially mirrored/reversed):

BARBICAN   2001-2002

FANCY IN THE GARDEN

COSMIC

TREE

DOORWAY CAN ACTUALLY
BE WALKED THROUGH
USED IN STAGE PERFORMANCE
THEN INSTALLED IN ROOM
WITH POSSIBLE
VIDEO ELEMENT

SPIDER WEB

BEAUTIFUL
WOOD & CLAY
SCULPTED
DOORWAY

A.

C.

MIRROR

SHATTERED
MIRROR

FLOWERS OR
PENNIES OR
CLOTHES

concept

SELF EXPANSION
THE COSMIC
WHOLE - THIS

CARDS IN
DOORWAY

B.
Cards:
to be taken
of drawings
and information
@ Cosmic Tree
and its relation
to story of "Fancy"

DOORWAY TO "WAY"
wood - clay
flowers
branches

Elisa Jimenez
Working drawing for performance,
September 2001
Watercolour, pen and ink

Both a mirror and a doorway, both a
truth about the self and its reversal,
both aged and new, Jimenez's
construction is a portal to the
imaginary worlds she creates in her
performances and with her clothes.

High End Performance
Art Projekt
bag people, 2001
Digital video

Perfect companions. High End
satirizes our investment in
fashion objects as things with
a life of their own. The project
documents a trip in which
the shopping bags become
participants, sitting around
beach fires as if they were
on holiday together.

ancient ritual, seeks it as a site of seclusion, a
specifically feminine solipsism. By contrast,
just as her 'clothes' problematize the
boundary of fashion and art, Jimenez
destabilizes the nature-culture association,
her emphasis on feminine eroticism and the
import of the ritual into the urban, recalling
the specifically female, illicit but licensed,
and profoundly sexual festivals of classical
Greece, such as the Adonia.

In their shared insistence on a truth of the
sign, we might recognize a surprising
convergence of one aspect of feminist art –
profoundly at odds with the fiscal and
significatory economies of fashion – with the
logo-heavy message of the global, luxury
brand. Both insist upon an essential and
guaranteed truth, brought to bear upon the
body. If for Fleury the logo is understood as a
kind of prosthesis, both an attachment to the
body and and, as carried bag, a statement that
proceeds the act of wearing, which proclaims
itself to be the alpha and omega of meaning,
for essentialist feminism the body and the
earth are attached in a similar relation.
Jimenez, perhaps sharing Fleury's wariness
towards the sign but – since the body refused
by Fleury is precisely where Jimenez begins –
realizing it through wholly different strategies,

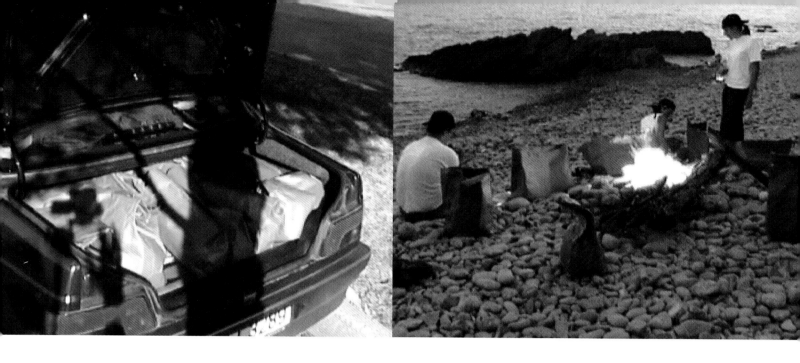

repeatedly subverts the absolute values attributed to fashion's signs. Indeed, we might say of Jimenez that rather than designing, she de-signs, insisting upon the body itself as prosthesis.

Jimenez's legibility as both designer and artist is recognizable only in the self-meditation of the wearer. In the graffiti 'signatures' of street-credibility commissioned by Marc Jacobs upon already authorized Louis Vuitton products, paralleling the signatures of graffiti artists where the 'tag' may constitute the entirety of the work (art residing in authorship rather than in its authorization), we have already seen how the guarantee of completion and individuality becomes a shared property of art and fashion. What of those who do not sign? Authority and authorship remain vested in the brush stroke, or *pace* Pollock, the dripped, the splashed, the thrown. The improvisatory gesture of the hand, the insistence on the specificity of the hand which made the mark, becomes the signature, the integrity of the work standing in for its guarantee.

Jimenez's partial shift to dressing the general body in select boutiques from the provisionality of 'sculpting' fabric on the specific body for specific wearers, necessitated a guarantee of her now absent authority. As Sarah Hailes of the SoHo store Kirna Zabête put it, 'I had to hand her a black Sharpie pen ... it was important to our customers to know they were buying the real thing.'[6] Jimenez signed the labels backwards, so that her mark, already tangible as a totality in the garment itself, only became readable in the context of self-awareness within the dress. If you weren't looking in a mirror, you didn't, apparently, know who'd made the garment. For Jimenez the dress was already signature, but it was effectively a mark produced by the body. The entire dress 'spoke' in the absence of its creator, but that articulation was only possible in the correspondence of dress to the wearer on whose body it had been designed. Jimenez's signature only became necessary in the absence of a specific body as much as in her absence as designer. This very different deployment of the logo – writing backwards, writing 'illegibly' – contrasts the two strategies that Fleury and Jimenez adopt in their resistance to the imposition of fashion on the body, the writing of the body through a logo-centrism. For Fleury there is a continual deferral, achieved through a signification out of context. The clothes never get to the body:

we see choice but never the inscription of another's language as consequence of that decision. Designed on, and to an extent with, the individual, we might understand the dresses of Jimenez's 'Hunger World' as at least as close as fashion, in its incoherent and dissimulating system of signs, can come to utterances in the first-person present tense. More than couture, where the design at least precedes the wearer, these garments assert individual identity. It is only in that assertion, or through the wearer's look in the mirror, that the absent designer is made manifest. Quite what Jimenez is signing her name to – a questionable truth of the body, and the veracity of the dress as statement about its model – is another matter entirely. 'The Hunger World' and the characters that peopled it, were fictional concepts. Wearing the costume one perhaps inhabits the contextualizing space of the artist's imagination rather than the exigencies of reality, and what may be 'true' in one world is not necessarily 'true' in another, nor even a practical guide to truth. The internal instability of the fashion object unfolds only through an ethical mobility of the sign ●

10

NOT CUT TO PATTERN

I WONDER WHAT SHE SEES. DOES SHE LIKE THE WAY SHE LOOKS?

Justine Picardie
'Creating Kate',
Vogue, May 2000

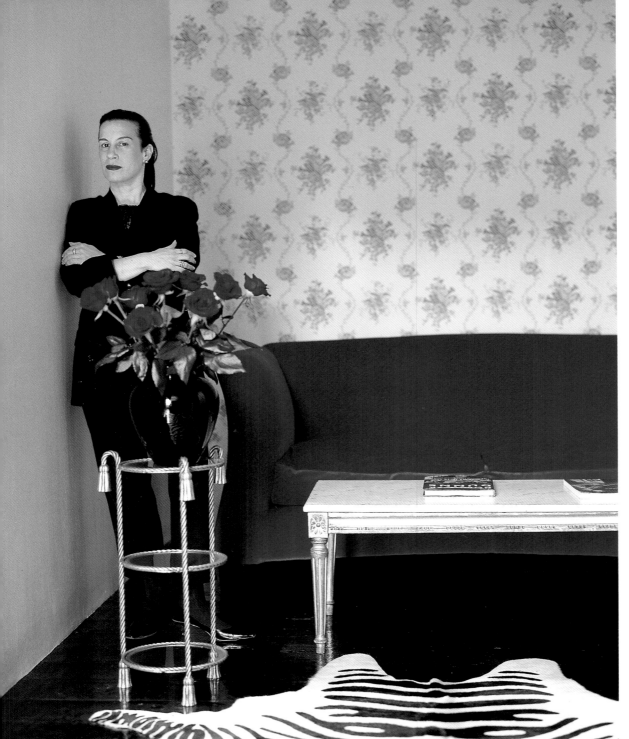

left
Edina van der Wyck
Maureen Paley
British *Vogue*, June 2000

The doyenne of East End
gallerists, with her artists –
Wolfgang Tillmans, Hannah
Starkey, Sarah Jones – in fashion
magazines as both practitioners
and subjects, becomes in turn
the object of fashion's attention.

opposite
Tracey Emin/Vivienne Westwood
Tracey Emin and Mat Collishaw
for Vivienne Westwood,
spring/summer 2001
Magazine advertisement

The face of Brit art becomes the
face of fashion. Emin's exposure
through press, television and
even, remarkably enough, her
art, makes her into a fashion icon
for a designer – Westwood – as
improvisational and idiosyncratic
as herself.

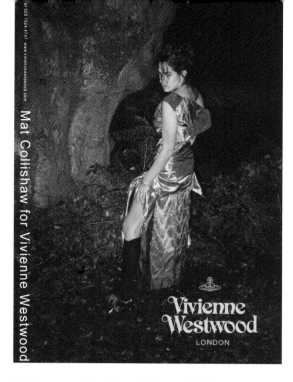

Mat Collishaw for Vivienne Westwood

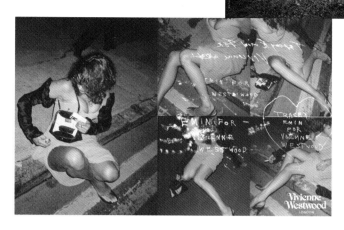

For the generation of (mostly) young British artists who came to be known, in art world shorthand, as the yBas, emerging from London and regional colleges in the late 1980s and early '90s, a straightforward critique of fashion, either as object *qua* object or as object of ideology, was never a consideration. Reacting to the aridity, inaccessibility and humourless expression of much of their tutors' art, the yBas were wary of over-intimate engagements with either political radicalism or theoretical explications in their work. Much of these artists' output would be described as 'conceptual', defined by a lineage running back to Marcel Duchamp via Bruce Nauman, but many of their rapidly developing oeuvres were profoundly object-based and their producers, in canny appreciations of art history, also seemed at times to systematically reiterate the public strategies of Warhol. For the yBas the notion of the artist as media darling was never a problem: the artist could critique a society of celebrity spectacle from within its architecture rather than erecting oppositional structures inside the sad cloisters of academia. Art and artists, reinstated as commodities, thus assumed higher profiles, using mass-media images and strategies, and moreover became relevant once more to the audiences of mass culture, even if critics rooted in mythologies of avant-garde radicalism failed to see it that way.[1]

The engagement with public curiosity that arose from well-publicized artwork and carefully promoted artists led to renewed interest in new art, not so much from fashion designers already cognisant of art and its histories, but from mainstream fashion magazines. Artists, as much as their work, became the subject of regular and extensive features. If art (not so suddenly but, nonetheless, surprisingly) was hip, it was necessarily a topic for regular debate – even if the framing of such discourse was usually limited to discussion of personalities rather than formal or ethical content. It was not only artists who were subjected to this treatment. Gallerists and dealers also emerged as fit subjects of inquiry: Jay Jopling, whose White Cube had become one of the principal commercial outlets for the yBas, cropped up regularly in society-page photographs, accompanied by his wife, the artist Sam Taylor-Wood.

With Interim Art, Maureen Paley had been a pioneer gallerist in London's East End long before it was thought fashionable as a location. In September 2000 Paley appeared in the 'My World' section of British *Vogue* – a single-page survey of a glamorous life normally reserved for models, jewelry designers and fashion celebrities. 'My World', of course, posed the kind of questions that no self-respecting art magazine could have asked, even if it had longed to. The interviewer never mentioned art, though Paley managed

to filter in her impressive roster of gallery artists, and identified the founding of Interim as the defining moment of her life. That was in 1984, a moment when no one in fashion's upper registers, least of all at *Vogue*, was paying much attention to cutting-edge art. If an unusual subject, Paley was perhaps a deserving one. Since her early years in London, contributing as a photographer to the second issue of *i-D*, Paley had remained engaged with the fashion world – an interest with important implications for certain of her younger artists. Furthermore, Paley's always immaculate and elegant personal appearance was in profound contrast to the dress codes of most yBas and their associates. Even if art permeated fashion magazines, most artists still dressed down rather than up, though perhaps now with a more deliberate excess and idiosyncrasy and greater self-consciousness. Sam Taylor-Wood was also amongst those prepared to insist on elegance, but perhaps the highest profile of art world 'fashionistas' was achieved by Tracey Emin.

Emin's rise to international fame looked more like the attainment of notoriety to the largely male critics who recoiled from a profoundly expressionist art articulated through the precepts of conceptualism. The public profile that accompanied the ill-informed media hullabaloo about carefully considered artworks such as *My Bed*, was, naturally, interesting to advertisers

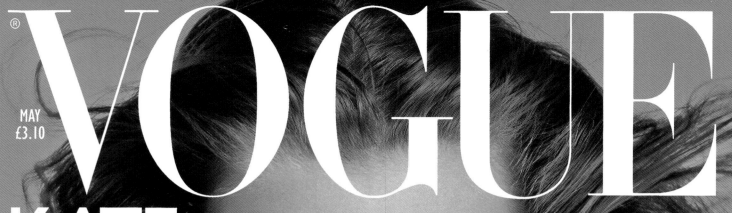

VOGUE

MAY
£3.10

KATE MOSS
SEVEN
GREAT
ARTISTS'
21ST CENTURY
MUSE

MARIO
TESTINO
SHOOTS
SUMMER'S
NEW
GLAMOUR

DOES
CHANGING
YOUR
BREASTS
CHANGE
YOUR
LIFE?

FASHION
MEETS ART

opposite
Sarah Morris
Kate Moss
British *Vogue* cover, May 2000

right
Sarah Morris
KTMSS, 2000
Gloss household paint on canvas

On the one side the archetypal fashion photograph: carefully lit, obsessively styled to remove any trace of naturalness and wholly conditioned by the model's seductive glance at the camera – and the spectator. On the other, a painting that obstructs the blatant readability of the photograph; a painting that reduces and reorders its components into the most basic building blocks of colour and shape, and leaves us with an almost abstract image, which we only understand as representation if we compare it to the original photograph.

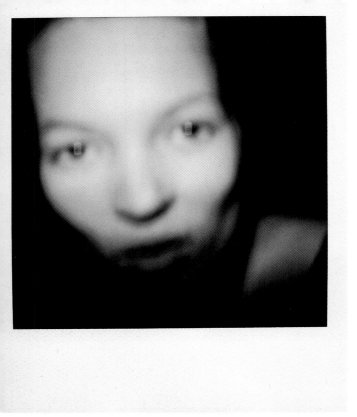

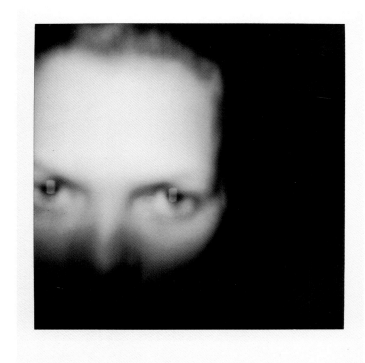

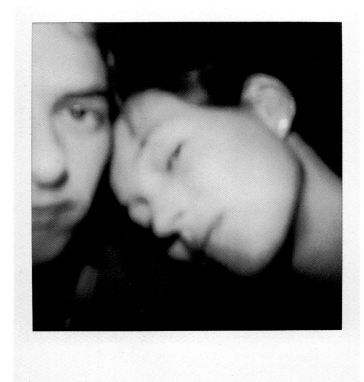

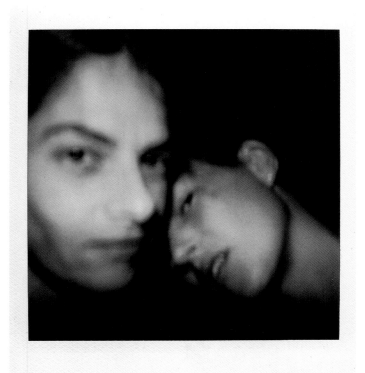

clockwise from top left
Tracey Emin
Mosskin, 2000
Polaroid photograph

Tracey Emin
Mosskin, 2000
Polaroid photograph

Tracey Emin
Tracey Emin + Kate Moss, 2000
Polaroid photograph

Tracey Emin
Tracey Emin + Kate Moss, 2000
Polaroid photograph

The intimate and everyday token of
ordinary friendship here becomes a
sign of intimacy between 'ordinary',
street-wise celebrities, and a signifier
of the embrace shared by art and
fashion at the end of the 1990s.

and marketeers. Emin was a recognizable figure, and face, with a strong constituency in a particularly affluent market. The artist also had certain clearly identifiable public traits. Her fondness for a drink led to invitations to appear in advertisements for spirits, whilst her panache in dressing was acknowledged by that former *eminence peroxide* of punk, Vivienne Westwood, who used Emin both as a catwalk model and in adverts. This relationship arose not simply because the artist could be deployed as a novelty marketing tool, but perhaps because the designer recognized in Emin's improvisational approach to dress – its visual strategies mirroring her way with materials in art – a spirit sharing the energy of the punk era. In Emin's work the quotidian was re-deployed as expressive object through a hand-crafted aesthetic, where earlier conceptualism had used it to arrest expression. Just as punk had shifted its register, in Emin's dressing her resistance to this intellectual policing was displaced onto the body.

Emin's special status, together with White Cube's high profile, would play a central role in one of the major projects that symptomized the close relationship, in Britain at least, between young artists and the fashion world. In January 2000 *Vogue* invited a number of leading yBas to collaborate with Kate Moss, producing new works which positioned the model as a '21st century muse'. American painter Sarah

Morris photographed Moss wearing Dolce & Gabbana for the cover of the May issue. Morris then digitally modified the image, gradually blocking its obvious 'readability', to produce a lambda print that in turn became the working model for a subsequent painting. Morris's work depended upon formal displacements between roles, those of fashion photographer and portrait painter, and media, specifically photography and painting, which also examined the accessibility of the image.

Emin's project with Moss, by contrast, explored the intimacy and rapport which was quickly established between the two women. Moss, since the earliest days of her modelling career, had often relied upon close relationships with particular photographers – notably Corinne Day, Nick Knight and Juergen Teller – who in turn depicted her in domestic and everyday surroundings. In such scenarios, Moss's body – our perceptions heightened by the history of her 'ordinary' South London origins – perhaps makes a spectacle of the everyday in much the same way as Emin, in constructing a spectacle of self-representation, relies upon the re-positioning of the domestic, the overlooked and even the abject. There is perhaps a commonality of moral panic between the reactions to Moss's 1991 *Vogue* shoot with Day, featuring an ordinary girl, in an ordinary room, in ordinary underwear, and Emin's

oeuvre, which proceeds not so much from phobias about particular depictions of young women or explicit autobiographies, as the presentation of the mundane as beautiful, truthful and worthy of attention. Body and art solicit scrutiny and pathos through a deliberate poverty: Moss beautiful by destabilizing conventional model agency measures of beauty, Emin meaningful, and at times 'beautiful', by expressing herself through the least expressive of materials.

Emin produced a series of Polaroids of Moss naked in the artist's bedroom, entitled *Mosskin* – an affectionate nickname, and also a play on the model's nudity. There is a resonance between these remarkably tender studies, the early work made by Corinne Day for *The Face* when Moss was still in her teens, and a more recent portfolio by Juergen Teller, which appeared in the relaunched *Nova* magazine. There Moss's nudity and posturing had deliberately mimed the exaggerated and stereotyped bodily dispositions and disclosures of pornography. In showing Moss as sexually alluring, Teller revealed the seductive properties that had fuelled her success as a model. T. J. Clark, writing of Manet's central figure in *A Bar at the Folies Bergères,* 1882, describes the young woman's visual impact as originating in part from 'a face whose character derives from its not being bourgeois and having that fact *almost* be hidden. For if one could not be bourgeois – if that status was always pushed

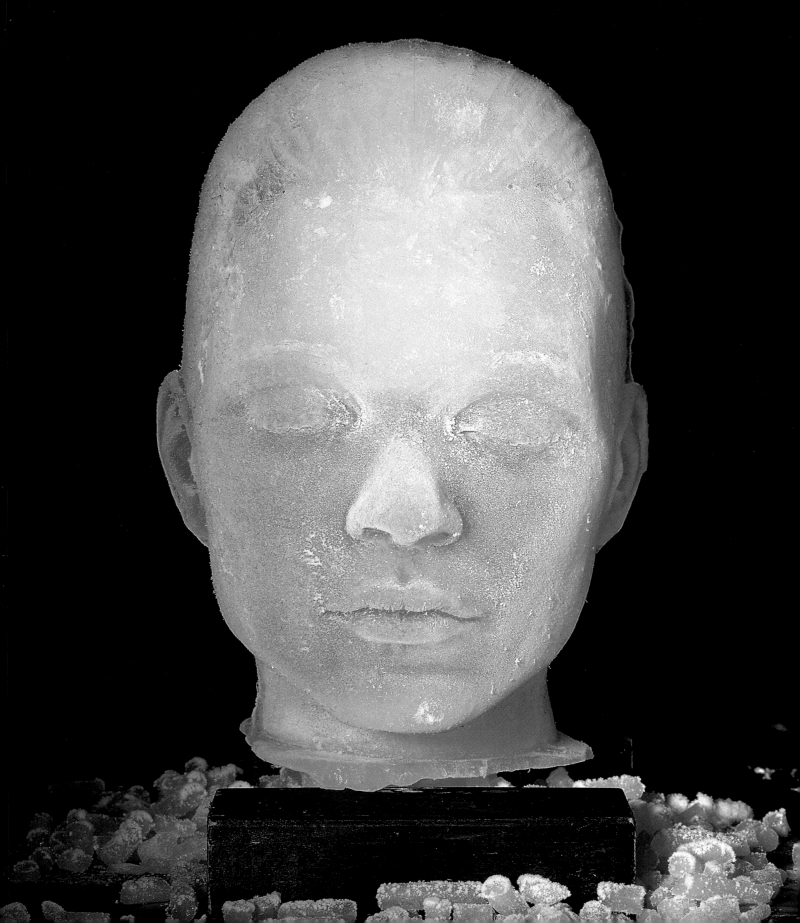

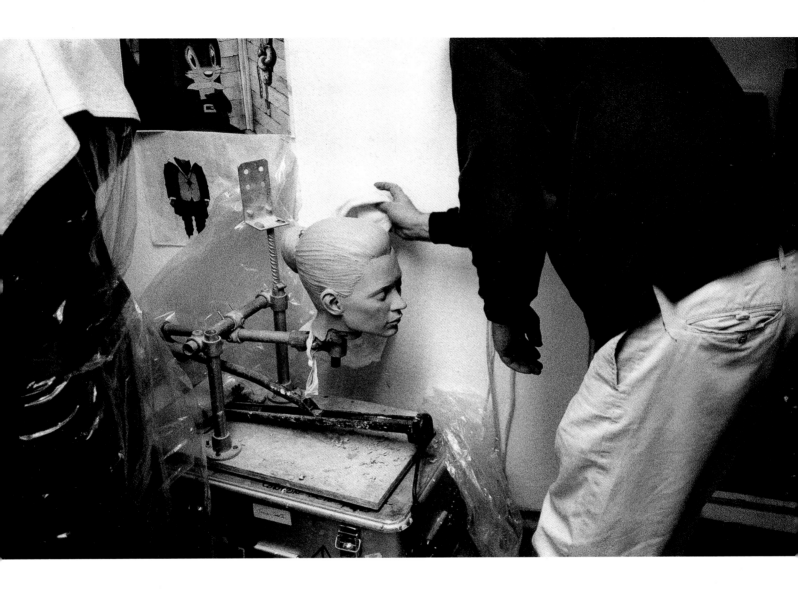

opposite
Marc Quinn
Study for *Beauty*, 2000
Stainless steel, glass, evaporating
frozen water, refrigerating
equipment

This is perhaps as real as the
fashion model gets; as close as we
may come to seeing and touching.
All that is solid melts into air.
What we imagine to be tangible
is proved to be intangible image.

above
Marc Quinn
Casting of *Beauty*, 2000

A process of transference: from body
to mould to plaster to ice ... to air.
Quinn's sculpture captures not only
the evanescence of a model's beauty
but the disposability, fragility and
artificiality of her representation.

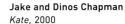

Jake and Dinos Chapman
Kate, 2000
Etching and watercolour

'Come up and see my etching...'
The decapitated self-portrait is
cast adrift in a cutesy cartoon
world where everyone else
is similarly bereft of a body.
The Chapman brothers spike
the pretensions of the fashion
world and parody its cruelty.

just a little further out of reach – then at least one could prevent oneself from being anything else: fashion and reserve would keep one's face from *any* identity.'[2] Hilton Als, writing in *The New Yorker* in the wake of Day's controversial portfolio, had understood similar qualities to be manifested in that work – a similar spectacle of downplayed difference, a similar opportunity for a muted bourgeois *nostalgie de la boue*, which Teller and Moss would exaggerate. Describing Moss as 'awkward, thin, disconsolate', Als outlined the lure of Day's 'vision of a young woman who was unaware of the corrosive effects of time as her soul rotted or played at the fringes of boredom, and unaware of anything remotely recognisable as "glamour"'. By over-emphasizing the quotidian as glamorous, Teller discloses the 'facts' whose partial occlusion/partial exposure made his subject such an alluring token of exoticism and difference for the fashion industry.

Emin's Polaroids are an instant expression of the pose before the camera; the fashion photographer's equivalent of a preparatory drawing, and perhaps a metaphor for Emin's own confessional, intimate discourse. In them, however, Emin seems to explore affinities between Moss's use in fashion of her own body (to the degree to which the model suggests its deployment rather than merely submits it to photographer and stylist) and the artist's own emphasis on

corporeality. Emin herself was no stranger to nudity. The performance *The Life Model Goes Mad*, 1996, had involved her living naked for a week in the space of a Stockholm gallery, whilst producing paintings and drawings. Much of that work took its stylistic lead from the work of Egon Schiele, even if its content, and Emin's performance, were ethical ripostes to the Viennese modernist's appropriations of hystericized, lubricious femininity. Emin's monoprints, similarly taking a stylistic leaf from Schiele's pad, nonetheless reversed – in both content and the practice of their making – Schiele's relationship to the sexualized, and often juvenile, thin, disconsolate, female body. The awkward, splayed and angular postures so quickly inscribed by Emin reflect those chosen by Moss and Teller for ironic presentation in *Nova*.

Marc Quinn's response to Moss's body seemed to share Emin's interest in autobiography. Best known for *Self*, 1991 – a cast of his own head, made with his own frozen blood – Quinn fitted Moss to a similar mould. The subject here, however, was the whole body, and the sculpture was realized with ice. Furthermore, Quinn chose to clothe the body, using an outfit supplied by Alexander McQueen, the young British designer closest to the yBas in both the trajectory of his public emergence and his temperament. Quinn's frequent recourse to refrigeration has emphasized the transitory

and perilous condition of his subjects, their permanence dependent upon external security and provision. The Moss sculpture further developed this theme. The immediate permanence that freezing offered was also responsible for the longer-term destruction of the subject. Over a three-month period the freezing process dehydrates the ice, slowly evaporating the solid so that it 'melts' into air.

As a commentary on the monumental, *Beauty*, 2000, uses fashion and the body in perhaps as knowing a subversion of sculptural conventions as the later work of Judith Shea. Quinn's monument – a single sign indexing, literally, in its casting from Moss's form, a singular body – must, to guarantee the necessary perpetuity of the monumental, be continually renewed. Rather than being a unique artwork, *Beauty* is a series that continually stages its own disappearance. The condition of monumentality thus corrodes, rather than affirms, its indexicality. That the subject of the sculpture is a well-known, attractive fashion model might lead us to understand Quinn's work as a commentary on the ephemerality of glamour and beauty. However, as *Beauty* vanishes beneath the effects of its own preservation, we could be looking at any ordinary, vulnerable body. The worn, fading solid ceases to equate itself to its absent index. Moss admitted herself to another form of vulnerability in a more hands-on

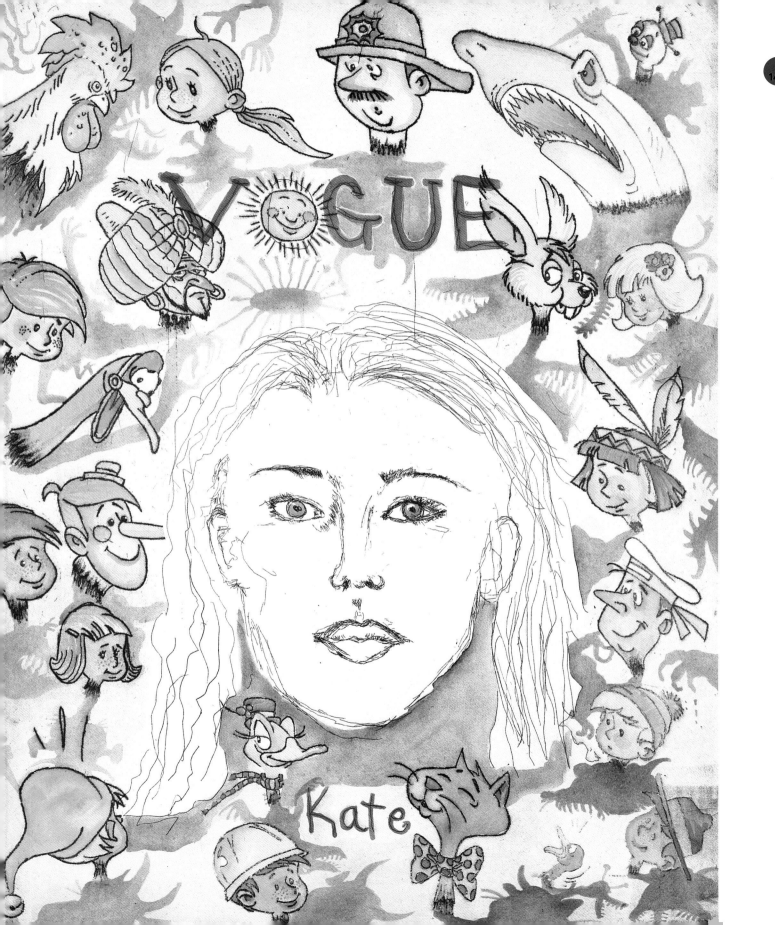

collaboration with the bad boys of British art,
Jake and Dinos Chapman. Reflecting their
interests both in utilizing the art of others
and in naïve art, the brothers set Moss to
work. The model, rather than modelling for
others, produced a model of herself – an
etched self-portrait which illustrates the
inflexible concentration and over-emphatic
line of the amateur artist. The Chapmans
then appropriated the etching, modifying
Moss's head and decorating the margins.
Uncannily, the pair produced a severed head
with disturbing resonances of Frank Moore's
portrait of Moss as Medusa (see pp. 6-7).
Both artists envisioned beauty as the subject
of violence – a theme we shall see repeated
and extended in much recent art that utilizes
and reflects on fashion.

The Chapmans further attenuated Moss's
already abbreviated autobiographical
statement, deploying it in their own fictional
world of distorted, victimized and lampooned
bodies. Moss looms like an intrusive alien
presence in a deliberately mutilated
cutesy cartoon world. We might read
in this iconography of disfigurement a
Chapmanesque critique of fashion and
celebrity: that Moss emerges as a figure
of the real in a comic-strip culture, and
that the sadism enacted against her self-
representation is a symbolic paralleling
of a cruelty perpetrated upon the model
in accommodating her to fashion's
prescriptions of the world. Moss had,

after all, been the victim of such a violence.
Emerging in the late 1980s, during the
second Summer of Love, as a signifier of
blissful (and blissed-out) youth in youth
culture's magazines, Moss's transformation
from aberrant waif to normative model had
been effected through a severance both
from that signifier's 'naturalness' and from
Corinne Day, the photographer to whom she
was closest, but whose insistence upon a
hard-edged realist vision was unacceptable
to many fashion editors. Increasingly,
both Moss's own life, and its mediated
representation in the cutesy cartoon world
of celebrity, was distanced from the 'reality'
of which she had been an icon. Through
the modification of Moss's self-portrait,
the Chapmans scrutinize the more general
diffusion of a 'local' youth culture into the
mainstream and question the agency of
the fashion model as volitional subject. The
etching perhaps suggests that here, in drawing
herself, and despite their intervention, Moss
has greater autonomy and expression than
she can be afforded by fashion.

Paradoxically, Corinne Day's exclusion
from high-end fashion magazines was
accompanied by an increasing dominance in
youth-market style magazines of a 'dirty-
realist' aesthetic, together with the
emergence of practising artists doubling as
fashion photographers. Fundamental to the
new generation of photographers and their
stylists were figures such as Larry Clark and

Nan Goldin. Goldin's pictures of a materially
impoverished but experientially rich
bohemian subculture, especially as portrayed
in her 1985 book *The Ballad of Sexual
Dependency*, provided a reference from which
young photographers took their bearings on
culture, and a romanticized vision of alterity
and exclusion with which young consumers
could empathize. The rejection of glamour
in British magazines in particular, including
The Face, *i-D* and the newly launched *Dazed
& Confused*, owed much to the look of Goldin
and Clark, together with a group of other
American artists such as Jim Goldberg,
Philip-Lorca diCorcia and Jack Pierson, who
featured in the artist-run magazine *ABeSea*.
By the end of the 1990s, the mutual interest
in, and collaboration with, the other's world
would lead to hybridized magazines such as
Pop – from the publishers of *The Face* – and
lower-budget productions such as *Made in
U.S.A.* and *Very* in New York. *Pop* featured a
wide selection of contemporary artists within
a slick lifestyle and fashion journal, and
demonstrated at least some appreciation
of the trajectory of art and fashion's
convergence by publishing recent work
from Duggie Fields.

Nan Goldin herself would take on some
projects as a fashion photographer – notably
for Helmut Lang and the Japanese retailer
Matsuda. The iconic status accorded to this
crossover perhaps exaggerated the
frequency with which the artist had moved

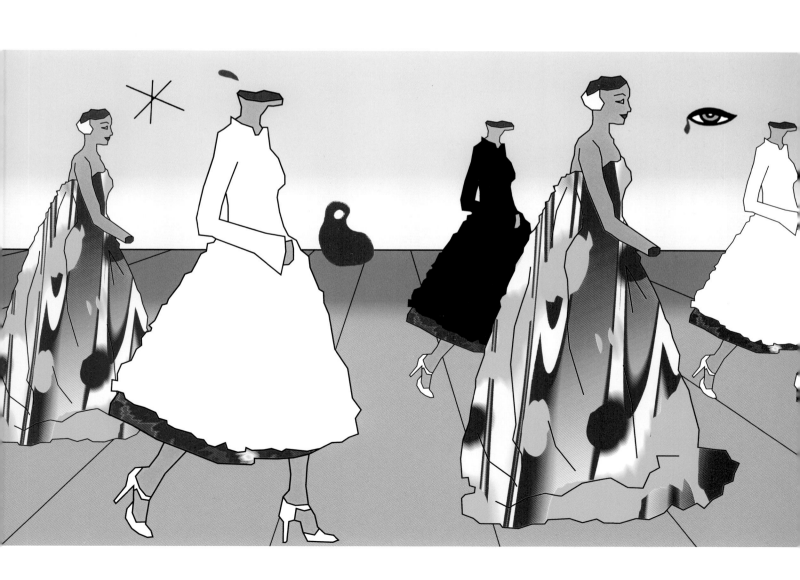

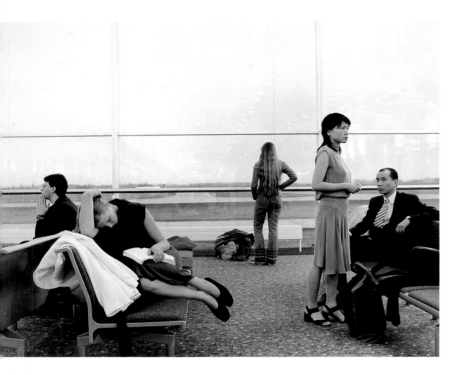

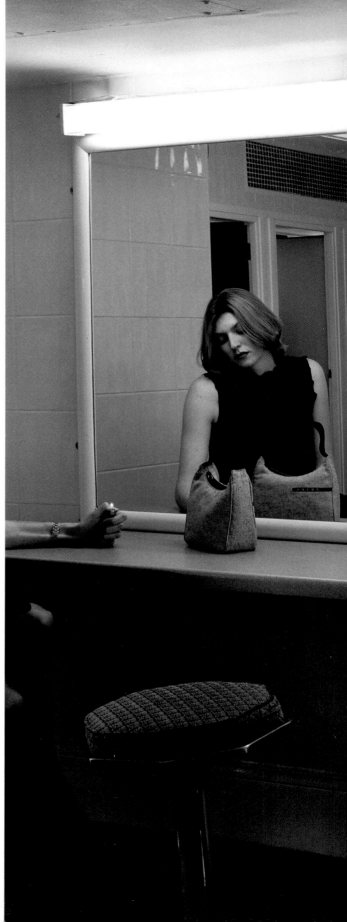

Hannah Starkey
Untitled – Vogue, August 1999, 1999
C-type print

There is a mutual prestige for
the parties in this situation.
The magazine shows off the latest
fashion through the latest art; the
artist is paid for appearing in a title
rather more prestigious than *Frieze*
or *Creative Camera*.

Hannah Starkey
Untitled – March 1999, 1999
C-type print

Ordinary people leading ordinary
lives. Starkey's studies of the
everyday are seamlessly translated
into fashion photography.
These could be large-scale images
in a gallery – eventually they
were – but they first appeared in
Vogue with captions identifying the
models' clothing.

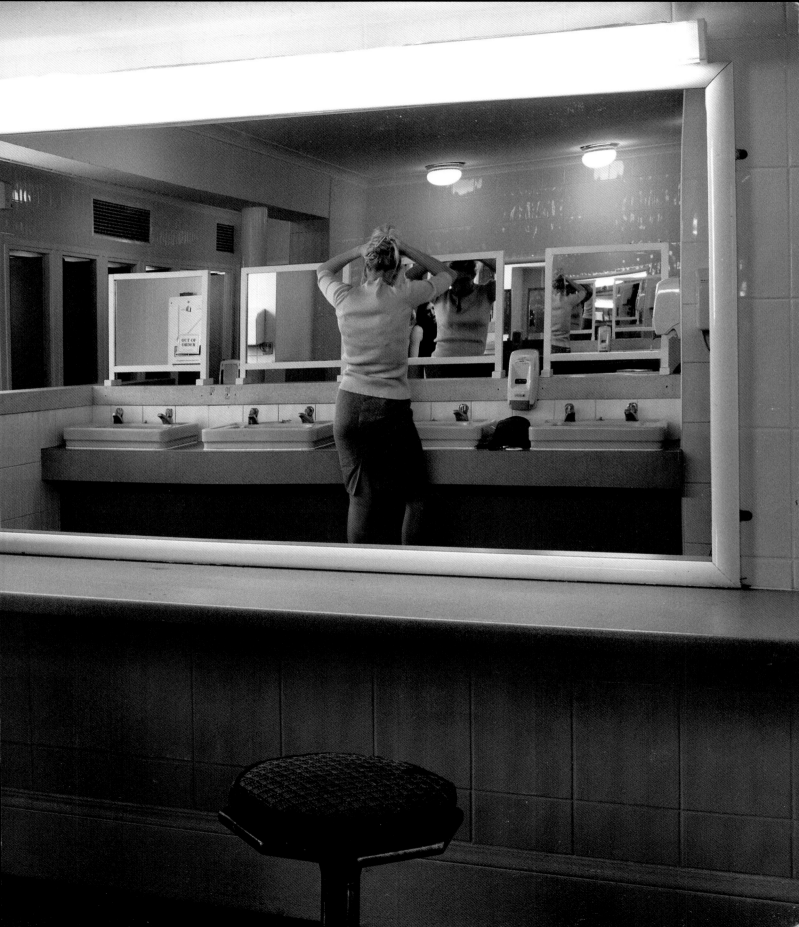

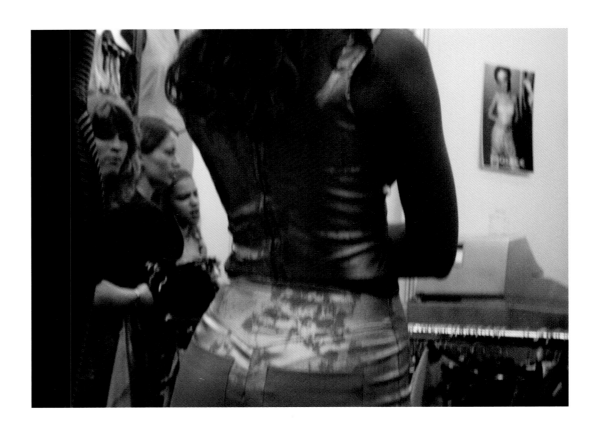

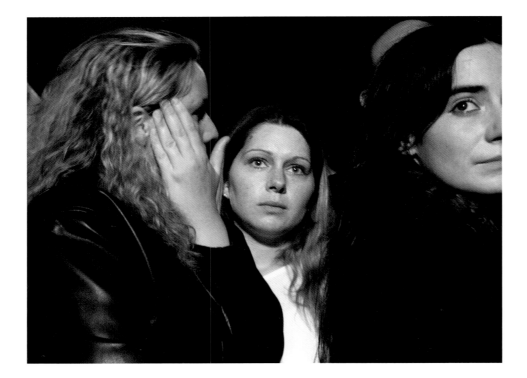

above
Henry Bond
Unique photograph *5012*, 2001
C print mounted using the
dyasec process

left
Henry Bond
Unique photograph *5021*, 2001
C print mounted using the
dyasec process

The casual glance of the camera
that mimics the informal fashion
photograph and captures the
everyday. In its haphazard approach
and attention to the ordinary, Bond's
imagery could be a critique of fashion
and consumerism. That it is
simultaneously both challenge and
endorsement is a provocation to
those critics who would have art fulfil
a political task, rather than exist for
the pleasure of the spectator.

Henry Bond
Unique photograph *5022,* 2001
C print mounted using the
dyasec process

Stories of the street. Bond's subjects
are too preoccupied with the everyday
to be composed and perfect as
models, yet they never stop trying
to be beautiful. Always in between,
they – even unconsciously – find a
split-second in which to pose.

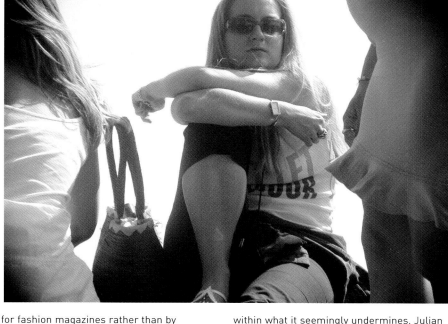

directly into fashion's orbit. Goldin's most
recent ventures into fashion magazines,
notably with French *Vogue* and British *Vogue*
(for whom she shot Kate Moss, styled by
Stella McCartney), have been as much a
platform from which to demonstrate
stylistic innovation and development as
to reprise her photo-history of the East
Village avant-garde. The transferability
between different activities of the artist's
role, and also of the style of work, is,
however, a notion that has been seized
upon by other artists and their gallerists.
The German photographer Wolfgang Tillmans
established much of his reputation within
fashion magazines, using the page spread as
a site of informal exhibition, and turning not
to the small-scale British art photography
press which was an accepted route for
artistic career development, but to the larger
circulation, mass-market journals of youth
culture. Maureen Paley, who encouraged
Tillmans from an early stage in his career,
was especially adept at helping her young
artists support themselves through work

for fashion magazines rather than by
simply selling artwork. Hannah Starkey, in
particular, demonstrated the permeability
of the once apparently solid barrier between
practices in a photo shoot for *Vogue.*
Starkey's images might have been
reproductions of prints exhibited in a show
at Interim Art: here, however, they were
commissioned by the magazine, used
professional models rather than the
amateurs with whom Starkey more regularly
worked, and were accompanied by captions
that identified the clothes those models wore.

Henry Bond's street-based projects, made
using a wide variety of cameras and media,
which evoked the fragmentary, constantly
disrupted visual experience of the modern
metropolis, seemed at times to take the 'bad-
image well-made' aesthetic of dirty-realist
fashion photography and return it to the
registers of fine art. Certainly there was much
about this work that recalled Impressionism,
not least Bond's emphasis upon the
provisionality and instability of the observing
gaze, reinforced by the artist's positioning
as a latter-day *flâneur,* and his attention to
subjects appearing to live lives more 'normal'
than the bohemian romanticizations of his
contemporaries. However, Bond occupies an
increasingly broad liminal domain between
fashion and art photography. Whilst his book
Cult of the Street could be read as 'a critique
of the aspiration of beauty',[3] alongside
subsequent enterprises it can also function

within what it seemingly undermines. Julian
Stallabrass clearly recognizes this in his
abrupt retreat from Bond's ambivalence into
fulmination – derived from the American
theorist Frederic Jameson – against the
'prison house of representation'. That Bond's
challenge to fashion and consumerism might
be simultaneously an endorsement of fashion
and consumerism, and therefore capable
of transformation into their promotion, is
demonstrated in a series of images for the
British fashion manufacturer Mulberry.
Rather than prolonging the agony of the
materialist insistence on the socially
transformative value of the art object,
the ubiquity of Bond's imagery demonstrates
the extent to which the yBa generation has
been prepared to re-invest in an art
premised upon pleasure. Even if many of
the objects that the yBas created were,
like Kate Moss, not conventionally 'beautiful',
a strategy for art's engagement with the
media and its audience emerged which
depended in large measure upon a similar,
limited revelation of difference as a source
of fascination. Such a strategy was inherently
adaptive, since it depended on the content
of the image itself rather than effects
presumed for the artwork but in fact
guaranteed by already established,
externally premised critical and political
agendas. Part of the pleasure, for artists,
as it had been for some time for makers of
fashion, lay in living with the contradictions
inherent in the objects of culture ●

11

TO DIE FOR

PERHAPS ART DEMANDS
THAT ONE PLAY WITH DEATH;
PERHAPS IT INTRODUCES
A GAME, A BIT OF PLAY
IN THE SITUATION THAT
NO LONGER ALLOWS FOR
TACTICS OR MASTERY

Maurice Blanchot
'Work and Death's Space'

Fashion plunges us into melancholy. Strange, that objects apparently so fascinating, so 'beautiful' – if only sometimes beautiful by difference from, rather than conformance to, conventions – so endlessly solicitous, so continually engaging in their recycling of novelty, should, in their estrangement from us, provoke introspection, violence, and demand an end. Which fashion suffers, now, at the hands of the artist. Seduced by the commodity, at a subjective level art perceives fashion's newness as originality rather than temporary placebo. Just as this dress, that suit, those shoes, will transform or complete us as individual subject to become last words, full stops on the sentences which articulate our selves. That is, of course, the condition that art imagines for itself. For almost three decades, with growing passion, artists have found in fashion's formal and thematic imaginations answers to the problems that art, having raised by interrogating its own language, by attenuating expression, could only ineffectually resolve. Recourse to fashion's thought and forms re-ordered the syntax of art, but at the same time it introduced new and vital elements. Now there emerges a realization that this vitality of language can be read like a death sentence; a pronouncement that, endlessly, in the violence of death, defers an ending and permits an infinite function for art. This is a realization that, like the always partial knowledge of infinitude, is profoundly unsettling.

A retributive, anxious violence is visited upon the object. We have been here before: with the disorder of Martha Rosler's collaged advertisements, re-ordering capitalism's announcements in the name of feminism; with Helmut Newton's victimized models in *The Story of Ohhh*; with Duggie Fields's

beautiful people – heads incised, limbs lopped. We have been here too in the more diffuse violence of refusal: the withdrawal from the thing into its concept, in the shift from looking into theorizing, in those phobic severances of the object of art from pleasure. Less this déjà vu seem too compact, too neatly reconciliatory of past to present, let us recognize that there is a dis-order to history, a flux, without the linearity or trajectory that invoking entropy might imply. Such recognizing blinds us to recognition: in the present we do not know where we are, even if its circumstances are familiar. We are always estranged from repetition. We have been 'here' before, but we do not know where 'here' is.

So in duplication, difference; in sameness, alienation; in the tangibility of things, an absence of essence. But with this folding of history, one era into another, there is subtle transformation. In the works of young artists responding to and exploiting our interest in fashion, just as violence is repeated so too the commodity repeats itself in seemingly novel forms. Art does not occult the savaged object; it exhibits the remains as spectacle. Art does not cleanly, incisively sever; it hacks and stabs, slashes, slits and tears. The tools and techniques of the serial killer and the Dada artist are imaginatively deployed upon the fashion object – magazine, model, dress – and rather than secret away the action of hate, despair or infatuation, what's left is hung with love for our appalled delectation. Sometimes these images have the literal look of the horrific cinematic. Izima Kaoru's

'murdered' models, the image of their deaths too colour-saturated and insufficiently prosaic to be documentary, are stripped filmically, wearing the designer clothes in which they have chosen to be 'killed'. The exhibition, these photographs' making permanent the moment, is a screen before disposal and decay – if they were only documents, before the bodies' resurrections – because they are desired fictions. Such a spectacle of violence has the effect, however, of memorializing, of making memorable the transitory. In Renaissance Europe the painted portrait emerged in part as a souvenir of the departed, its subject depicted not in the fact of death but as imagined in life. Photography – supreme memento mori – begins with the identical premise.

Kirsten Glass proceeds from the spectacle of ephemera that is the fashion magazine, from the stunning photographic image to which we never give a second glance. The drop-dead gorgeous drops dead; no one sees. Indeed, an absence of scrutiny is the cause of fashion death: wraith models fading into invisibility through neglect, walking in and out of each other's bodies and each other's times like the intersecting, overlapping catwalks of Silvia Kolbowski's video. The photograph, which should be the arrest of death, the stopping of the moment, guarantees mortality, inhumation, forgetfulness. As coding of the body it is too easy to circumnavigate, too easy to read presence as absence. The only way to resist your being forgotten: pose for another photograph until, as Siegfried Kracauer suggests, memory is heaped in a garbage dump of imagery and anonymous, captive time.[1]

Glass obfuscates this disposable transparency. Her principle is the collage: a scything through of mass-market magazines, a harvesting of glamorous figures. Her purpose in reusing the mass image is its revivification. The violence of

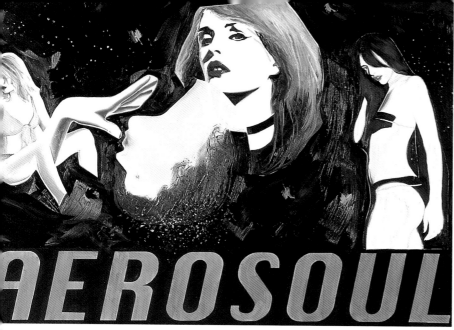

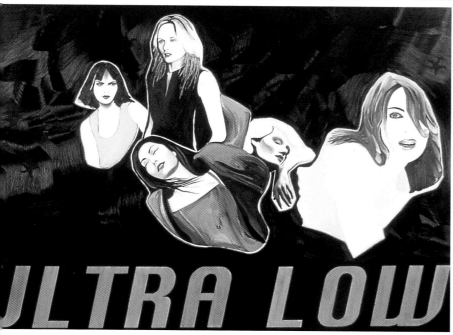

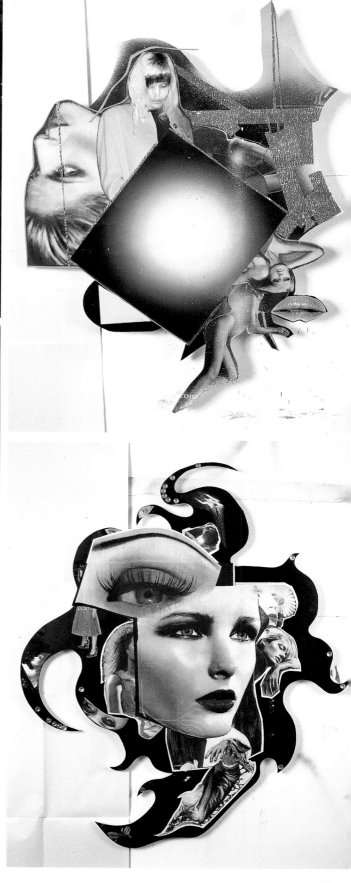

top
Kirsten Glass
Aerosoul, 2000
Oil on canvas

top right
Kirsten Glass
D. J. L., 2001
Mixed media collage

above
Kirsten Glass
Ultra Low, 2000
Oil on canvas

right
Kirsten Glass
Christine, 2001
Mixed media collage

Glass collages and reuses the mass-market image. For her paintings she creates enlarged photographic stencils, blowing up the fashion magazine to the scale of the billboard. In transferring its images to oil and acrylic, she overwrites the photograph's original meanings.

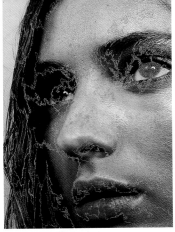

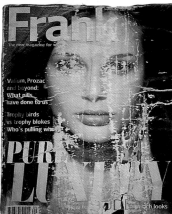

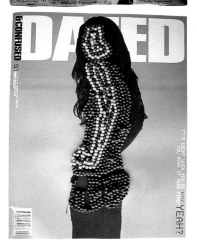

Frank
The new magazine for women

Valium, Prozac
and beyond:
What pills
have done to us

Trophy birds
vs trophy blokes
Who's pulling who

PURE
LUXURY

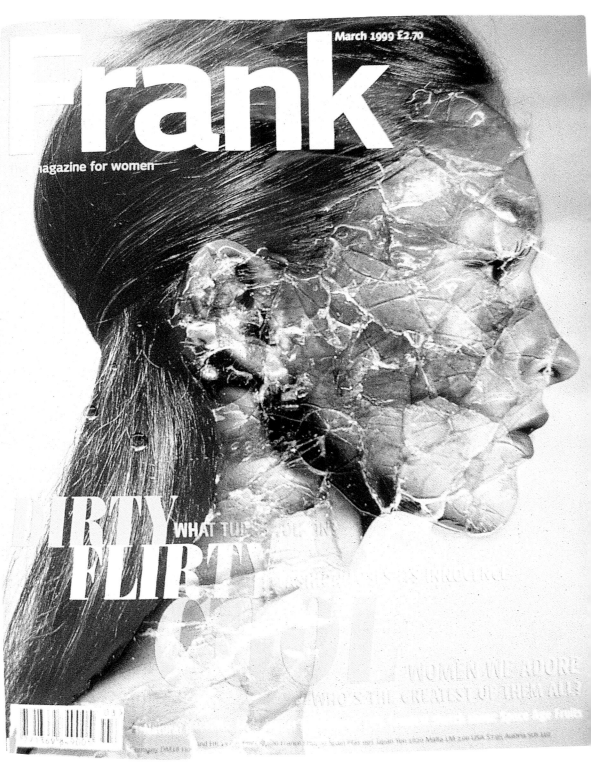

March 1999 £2.70

Frank

magazine for women

DIRTY
FLIRTY
WHAT TUR

WOMEN WE ADORE
WHO'S THE GREATEST OF THEM ALL?

collage yields a mobility of figure and meaning that escapes the petrification of time, putrefaction of memory, the photograph's encryption of a corpse. Glass's medium is generic confusion – is collage, is photography, is painting. Surgically knifed from context, the model's figure is re-photographed and blown-up as photographic stencil. Returned to the studio in this new form, the ghost of fashion's past is recirculated in a fluidity of paint. The instability of the reproductive medium resists the fixed intent of the photograph. An image of commodity or celebrity – which amounts to the same thing – whose first intent was to communicate the fact of that object, embodied within a network of potential identifications and personal meanings, is displaced into another temporal register, another regime of visual scrutiny. Rather than emptying the sign of meaning, Glass overwrites it, creating a double inscription, where one text occludes the other. Without naming names, for the identities of her subjects are, for now, mostly obvious to us, Glass retitles the receding, singular moment. Painted out of life, these fashion models and actresses escape the time of temporary identification. Art continues to suggest that the momentary, no matter how good, is nothing special until we know where, and when, it ends.

Blanchot, writing about Rilke, remarked on the poet's anguish at anonymous mortality. 'One doesn't want to die just anybody's undistinguished death. Contempt for anonymous disappearance, for the "They die", is the disguised anguish to which the anonymous character of death gives rise.'[2] It is this anguish that Glass coolly articulates in her paintings, and this anguish that arises from a fundamental difference of art and fashion in the temporal structure – the duration – of their objects. No matter how close the two discourses come, no matter how intimate their coupling, Glass's violence upon the model exposes this incommensurability. As Barthes, Bazin and Metz persistently remind us, in arresting the passing moment the photograph is a kind of death. The fashion photograph – that massively costly investment of artist, model, stylist, hairdresser, make-up artist, location finder and assistants, recouped only in the instantaneous, low-cost encounters of the mass audience – is death heaped upon death. The image and its subjects are both ubiquitous and utterly disposable.

So too, notwithstanding a growing taste for retro, is the fashion object. Fashion and art may both recycle and resurrect their histories, but fashion re-makes its objects: it only rarely refreshes and exhibits the object of history as historical object (though Valentino's strategy of numbering and releasing garments from its archives is an exception). Diane von Furstenberg caused a minor sensation when she exactly reproduced in 2001 the very first linked-print wrap dress she had sent down the runway in 1972, accompanying the relaunch with the advert made to sell the garment nearly thirty years before. Such strategies remain rare, and might be considered the belated remaking of a concept or pattern – akin to the periodic, and historically different,

materializations of the instructions that constitute much of Fluxus art. The museum, now including much of fashion's archive, remains art's domain. Despite a growing taste for the contemporary and the immediate, art remains fixed upon retrospection and endurance. No matter how closely concerned with the disposable pleasures of commodity culture are, say, a Koons or a Rosenquist, those paintings will still be on display, valued long after their subjects are decomposing in the city dump. The reiteration of a limited range of expressive strategies might give rise to Neo-Dada, Neo-Expressionism, even to Neo-Pop, but alongside the new is exhibited the old, the object of the past sustained or at least rediscovered in the present, very often precisely as a context in which we come to understand the contemporary. Fashion, insistent upon the moment even in its rediscoveries, is less willing to mix and match styles or the histories that accompany them. History – for fashion – is best understood only through the all-consuming filter of the present. It is this changed context into which Kirsten Glass hauls her subjects, their transformation made more obvious as painterliness – an emphasis on gesture – develops in the young artist's oeuvre. Appropriated to the painterly commodity, the model becomes, with a resonance of Glass's own titles:

SOMETHING   ELSE

Art includes its own reiteration here. Where Glass lifts the image directly from the photograph, Duggie Fields drew and then painted the pose. Both preserve by

opposite top
Graham Dolphin
Untitled (soldering iron drawing 27),
2000
Magazine page burnt with
soldering iron

opposite centre
Graham Dolphin
Untitled (Frank, September 1998),
1999
Magazine soaked in bleach for
one month and then dried

opposite below
Graham Dolphin
*Untitled (Dazed & Confused,
February 1999 – pinned)*, 2000
Magazine, map pins

Each torn fragment a facet of a
complex identity smoothed over by
fashion's unguents. Moisturizing, for
Dolphin, is certainly not the answer.

opposite main picture
Graham Dolphin
Untitled (Frank, March 1999 – resin),
2000
Magazine coated in resin
and smashed

A deliberate and gratuitous sadism
enacted with all the glee and
improvisatory wit of the fictional
serial killer. Dolphin solders a
displaced sketch of the model's
image over this month's version
of the perfect face.

Izima Kaoru
Kojima Hijiri wears Yohji
Yamamoto 231–233, 1999
Cibachrome

A fantasy of violent, glamorous
death, with high fashion as a vital
element in the ultimate final
performance for the world. It is
a transgression that extends
fashion's refusal of safety and
domestication to its most
extreme limit.

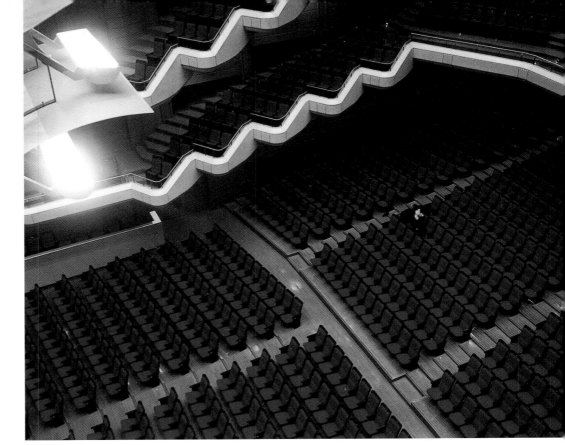

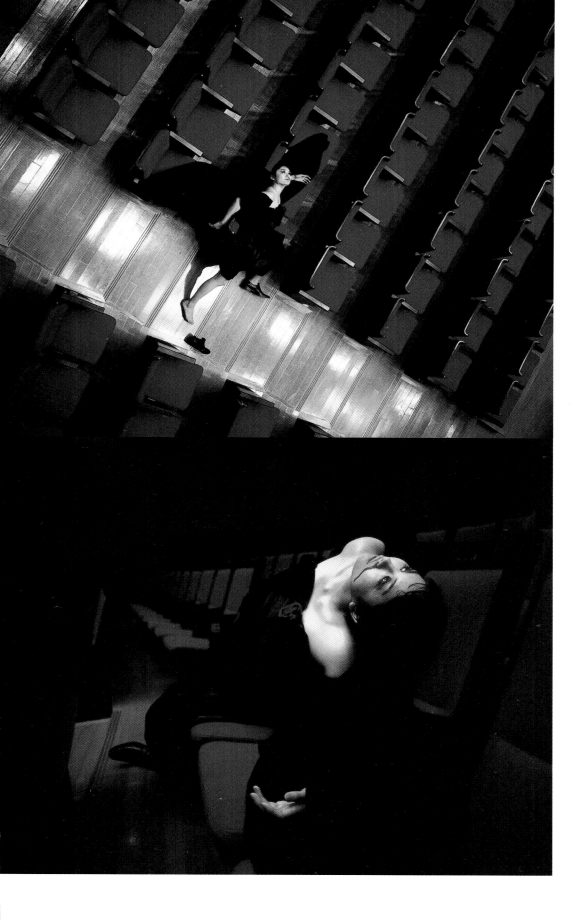

translating fashion's death into a new medium. Who now remembers the '70s? Who would turn back pages to the shoots that Fields took as his guides? Art holds the position that fashion abandons. Both Fields and Glass remain intrigued by the subject of their aggression. It is perhaps love at the heart of this violence, the desire to preserve, whereas more overtly political collagists exacted a toll of disgust and loathing, cutting to expose the horror, as they saw it, of the commodity's inner truth. Glass and Fields seem to suggest that at least half the truth of the commodity is what you paint into it.

Who now remembers the '70s? Perhaps – in a way learned through television, video and magazines – Graham Dolphin. The often extreme, sometimes witty violence he inflicts upon innocent magazine covers and their model subjects recalls the gratuitous viciousness of the early slasher movie. The first point of reference is perhaps a film as sadistic as *The Toolbox Murders*. Dolphin reaches repeatedly for the appropriate instrument of torture or dispatch: drooling solder over sensitive skin, impaling a model's face with a precisely measured grid of nails, substituting pins, bristling outwards, for Linda Evangelista's eyebrows and lashes, masking Christy Turlington's immaculate complexion with photo-mount, sealing the lips and leaving only the mute, residual eyes to communicate.

Dolphin perhaps exemplifies a paradigm of aggression and frustration that derives from the inadequate transferability of art and fashion's objects – hampered by the temporal differences that Glass highlights – and also from the incommensurability of each practice's internal discourses. The substitutive objects of an art made melancholy by fashion's continual necessary losses are not only artworks but also fashion objects which are as near to fashion as art can get. Fashion, however, remains intangible: it promises satisfactions it never provides. That the two discourses cannot ultimately converge because of fashion's endless deferral of the real, provokes, in Dolphin's art, an insistence on art's superiority through the stability of its objects and their discourses. The magazines that Dolphin attacks are not in themselves 'fashion'; they are, rather, surrogates for its slippage, its absence, which allow us to imagine what fashion is, but do not themselves constitute it (an instability that is, of course, fashion's aspiration as transitory object, and art's phobia,

projected, protected, in its determination of boundaries). Confronted with the inadequate communication of fashion's objects, Dolphin's response is to negate that flawed, perpetual signification with his own imposition of limit. His violence against the visual pleasure of the object – fashion's primary tool amongst seductive ploys – is as much formal blocking and containment of meaning as it is a revenge attack upon the commodity and paradigms of beauty. From here the nails look like a holding in place, the glue mask an attempt at bonding permanently to one statement. Where Glass's over-writing of the signifier establishes palimpsests of meaning, Dolphin's is effectively an assertion of art's primacy, its right to speak in the place of the commodity. When he substitutes pills for the model's body, leaving only intimations enough to know that figure's place in the frame of fashion, Dolphin obliterates fashion's language and wholly privileges his – the artist's – own commentary. Art, here, is both fashion's poison and its cure; its pharmacy.

'Death, if it arrived at the time we choose, would be an apotheosis of the *instant...*'[3] The consciously posed photograph, the consent to arrest, might in its instantaneity be such a moment as Blanchot describes. Dead, the models in Izima Kaoru's images fantasize both mode and moment of dispatch, order the high fashion appropriate to such violent elimination. Photographed, they rise, wash off the synthetic gore, the mud and sand, and live, never again so perfect as in the dream of their destruction. Glamour, it seems, solicits a deadly violence, and violence demands glamour.

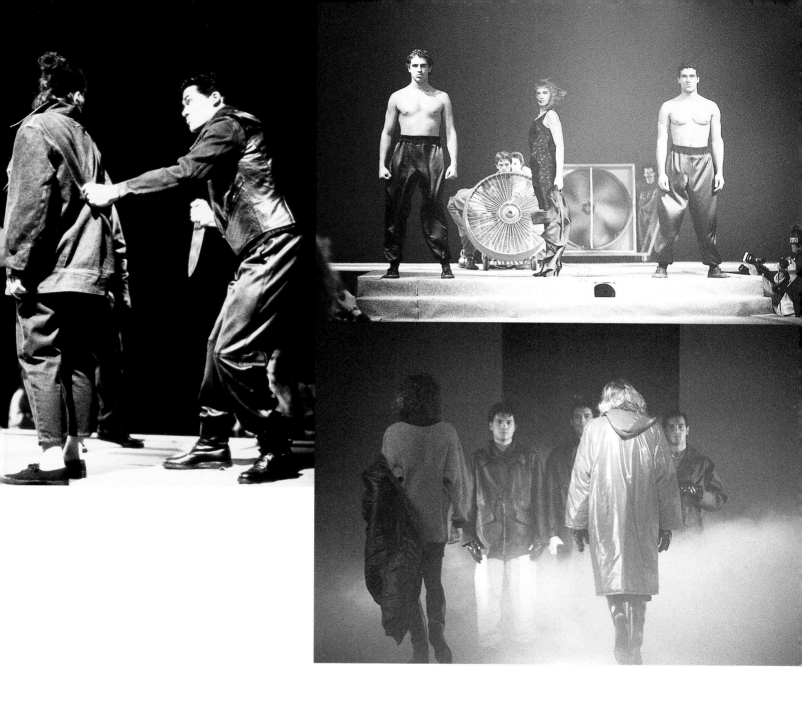

Dario Argento (director)
Fashion show for Trussardi Action,
9 March 1986

Death rendered preposterously
beautiful and glamorous; the fantasy
of cinema reworked as a lumbering
theatre. Horror film director Dario
Argento transposes moments from
his *Suspiria* onto the catwalk – the
models stabbed and dragged off-
stage in body bags.

In *Kojima Hijiri wears Yohji Yamamoto*, 1999, Kaoru takes us to that most opulent of cultural settings, the opera house, and disposes the model over the upper stalls. In three images he gradually closes in on the dead body. The first panel offers us context, a lush and empty theatre, and enigma, a residual figure, its posture awkward, shoulders bared, head thrown back. The sense of the cinematic is reinforced by the second panel: an overhead shot, as if a craned camera had overlooked Hijiri. We begin now to see details: one shoe slipped off, arms splayed out, torso twisted broken-backed across the plush upholstery. The figure appears like a stain on the ordered ranks of empty seating, an intrusion upon a tranquil and perfect emptiness. In its torsion there is something about the body that defies the camera's mechanically imposed perspective. The seats 'read' one way, the body another, as if it were an anamorphic trick that could only be resolved by viewing from a particular angle. That sense of stain, of both subject and spectator being out of order and out of place, is reinforced by Kaoru's use of shadow and the spread of fabric from the Yamamoto gown. The umbral folds and claret silk resonate with the rhythmic colour regime of seat and space, seat and space, and also disrupt their regular pattern. In the final image of the sequence, Kaoru, shooting now close-to and low-down, emphasizes these shadows yet more effectively, so that Hijiri's bare flesh – shoulders and head, an isolated

hand – seems fragmentary and disconnected from its setting. The dress emerges from and disappears into the darkness of the theatre, its 'stage' suddenly darkened. The head, turned back, eyes opened, looks back in an empty gaze at the balcony from which the body has plummeted. A trickle of blood across the face picks up the deep red of the seating and directs our attention to a just-highlighted whorl of cloth in the 'dead' woman's décolletage. The left hand, held open as if still pleading aid or attention, is rendered disproportionate through another anamorphosis – the gesture, oddly juxtaposed to the body's alignment, seems to belong to another time and space.

Kaoru's settings are fantasies, and most often fantastical. We do not anticipate our own murder, we do not select designer outfits in which to be killed, though we might in committing suicide – which is how many of these images could be understood. Violence in these pictures is volitional, and the excess of violence seems to answer an excessive glamour. It proceeds from fashion's emphasis upon, rather than domestication of, desire. Kaoru, who began his career as a fashion photographer, returns to the terrain inhabited by Newton and mapped out by Rosetta Brooks in *ZG* in the early 1980s. Indeed, Kaoru's pictures might be fashion photographs, innovations in a genre that thrives on continual transgression. The mise-en-scène in *Kojima Hijiri wears Yohji Yamamoto* has a profound resonance with Dario Argento's film *Opera*, 1987 – another exercise in conflating beauty, opulence, desire and death. And it was Argento who, a year after that film, also brought 'death' to the catwalk, directing a show for Italian manufacturer Trussardi in which he replayed one of his earlier films. 'On a catwalk, to the music of Pino Donaggio's *Body Double*, Argento recreated the opening moments of *Suspiria*, complete with rainstorm, and had the glamorous models stabbed to death, then elegantly carted off in see-through body bags.'[4]

The extreme and often bizarre violence visited upon Kaoru's models – witness *Akikawa Risa wears Chanel*, 1994, stabbed with scissors and rammed through the back of a sofa as if its upholstery were the boundary of before and after lives – parallels the frenzy of Argento's or Jesus Franco's aggression against bodies that are predominantly female. But in Kaoru's artful treatment of fashion's norms, there is, as Oosima Hirosi observes, a folding and a reiteration. Rather than breaking with convention, Kaoru turns it around and upon itself.[5] This is not simply a matter of incorporating cinematic horror, of glamorizing the scene of brutal crime. Hirosi remarks that 'Death is just one frame in the film of life, just a brisk walk through the city...'[6] and what Kaoru's series perhaps repeats, shifting register and scale, are the concerns of Robert Longo's late 1970s and early '80s work *Men in the Cities*. Longo depicted, in oversized drawings, young Manhattanites in frozen postures of dying. Those pictures were based upon Polaroids, posed by models, and their extrapolation of the pose into a protracted, hand-crafted economy is perhaps akin to Kirsten Glass's revivifications of the photographic dead. Of more relevance to Kaoru is the interpolation of Longo's work into fashion's imagery, co-opted by David James, styling a shoot by Phil Poynter in 1996 for a Japanese menswear catalogue, and employed by Juergen Teller in a campaign for Jigsaw menswear in 1997. The arrested posture of urban death is understood as another recognizable pose with which the spectator can identify. Longo and Kaoru both highlight death as condition of the urban experience; Kaoru adds that it is a necessary correlative of desire. Roland Hagenberg, writing on Kaoru, invokes his own testimony as victim

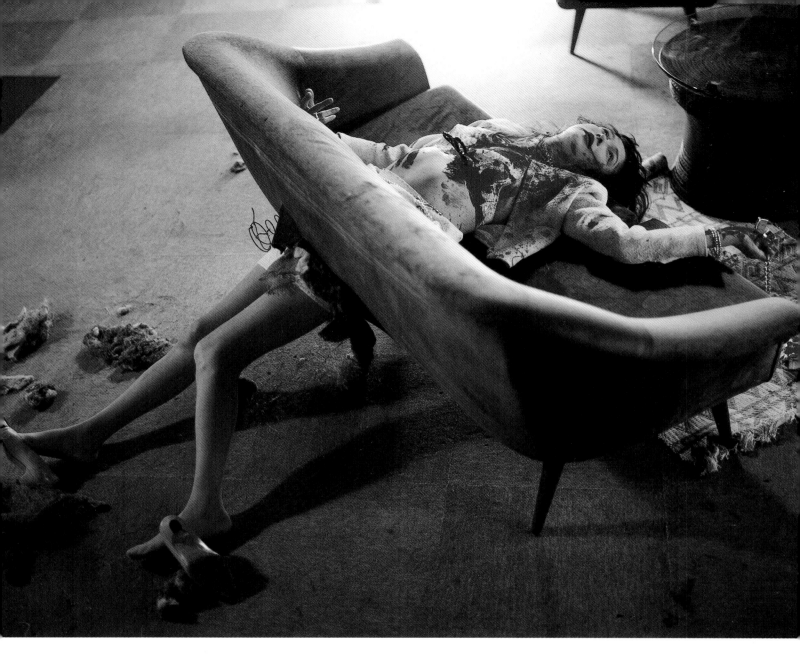

Izima Kaoru
Akikawa Risa wears Chanel 021,
1994
Cibachrome

An extreme and bizarre violence
wished upon the self – a making
into spectacle of which fashion
is a necessary part. If a Chanel
outfit is 'to die for', what more can
we do than choose to die in it?

of urban terrorism – being bombed by Basque separatists – and comments succinctly that 'life's versions of dying are mostly less elaborate'.[7] Like dying, however prepared or unprepared we are, life is less elaborate than our dreams. Fashion is a hyperbolization of desire, not its negation; art, too, a manner of making experience particular. Even up to and including violent death. That sadism and desire might indeed be vectors of everyday experience which fashion highlights, and indeed draws us towards, rather than a combination to be avoided, is illustrated in Kaoru's recent *Helena Noguerra wears Vivienne Westwood*, 2001, based upon a fantasy of its model's death games with her husband, pushed both a step too far and to their desired limit.

At the conclusion of Georgina Starr's performance (and subsequent DVD installation) *The Bunny Lake Collection*, 2000, dead models in shimmering silver gowns lie heaped upon a catwalk. Bloodstains spread over the fabric from gunshot wounds. Assassinated by children, rather than offering only a voyeuristic memory as they finally disappear backstage, these models leave a beautiful corpse behind. Starr's piece can be read as a multi-layered commentary on both art and fashion's relationship and fashion's impact upon the individual. That the killers here are children rather than the malevolent stalkers of Argento's catwalk staging for Trussardi suggests a resistance of innocence to the sophistication and sexuality that the glamorous gowns suggest. These murders look like the imaginary aggression of the child against the adult world; refusals of what the little girls, so inappropriately equipped with automatics, are supposed to become. The young girl represents the world of the imaginary – where identity is misunderstood as unbounded and autonomous – in contrast to the symbolic value of the woman on the catwalk, where the fully sexualized and fetishized figure is presented as an object of attention in the gaze of others, and perhaps only exists through it. If childhood is an imaginary, naïve freedom, adulthood, for all

its seductive promises of sophistication, is a captivity in which the individual is no longer capable of real expression. The dress of the first model on the catwalk bears the embroidered legend 'She is alive'. Starr's response seems to be both 'Not for long!' and 'Prove it! (by dying)'.

In its brutally simple, convergent narrative – we should not forget that amongst Starr's most impressive work is the cartoon strip *Tuberama – The Bunny Lake Collection* offers both a model of the individual's relationship to fashion as a figure of maturity, and a mocking commentary on the fashion world itself. The little girls run through the streets towards their carefully plotted act of assassination, as age would carry them towards the sexualized maturity that the fashion show represents. Meanwhile the models parade up and down on the catwalk, going nowhere. For all its claims to avant-garde status and the promise of constant progress, fashion is depicted here as locked into a kind of stasis, a self-conscious walking on the spot. Starr's judicious use of low camera angles, shooting upwards from the level of the catwalk, establishes the models as rather pompous and slightly ridiculous. The catwalk show ends not in the usual triumph but in carnage as the girls open fire. Starr synchronizes the muzzle flashes of guns to a larger, syncopated rhythm of flashing light, as if the show's designer had chosen to end the display with a flicker effect. Staging mimes the effect of gunfire and, crucially, the flashes of cameras from the photographers beside the catwalk. In fashion, Starr seems to be suggesting, it doesn't matter how you get shot – with gun or camera – just as long as you make a

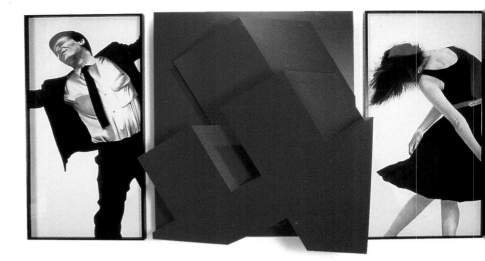

Robert Longo
 # 41 Untitled, 1982–4
Mixed media

'Death is ... just a brisk walk through the city.' Longo's drawings distil a particularly urban paranoia about the violence that seems an inescapable part of metropolitan life.

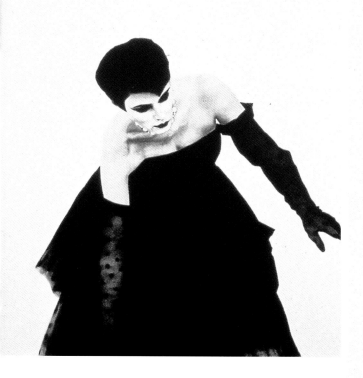

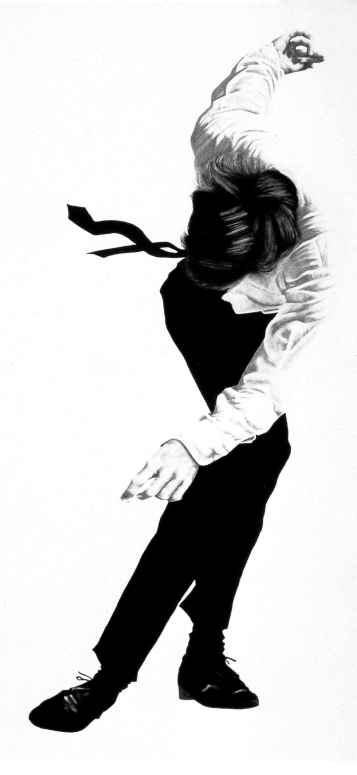

above
Robert Longo
D-12 Untitled, 1980
Charcoal and graphite on paper

right
Robert Longo
D-53 Untitled, 1981
Charcoal and graphite on paper

The poses and the costumes of Longo's victims, along with horror, promote a certain romanticism and idealism. Dying, everyone is fixed in heroic postures and perfect city clothes; everyone stays young. That romance is a source for fashion's use of these postures, these pictures. Just as young, paranoid urbanites of the 1980s could identify with the fate of Longo's subjects, so street-smart fashion victims can transfer their own fears, not onto art, but into what they might want to wear.

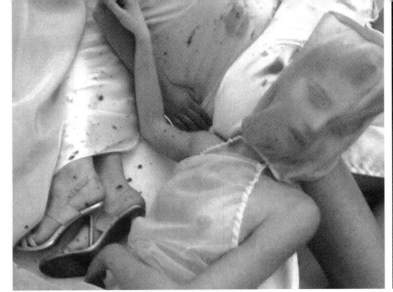

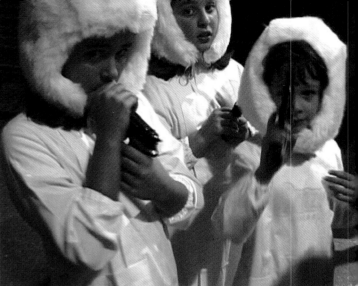

Georgina Starr
The Bunny Lake Collection, 2001
Selection from set of 16 C-print
photographs

An imaginary resistance to the
glamour and sexuality of the adult
world: Starr's infant killers take
revenge on the symbolic culture of
the catwalk and their future position
on it. The little girls' nihilism is an
expression of desire which maturity
would strip from them.

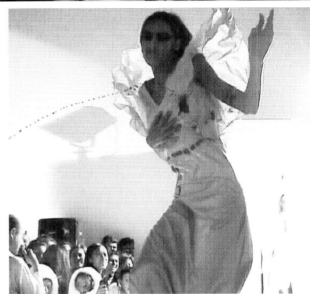

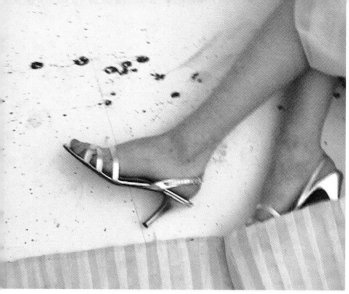
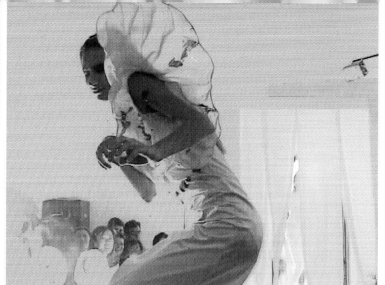
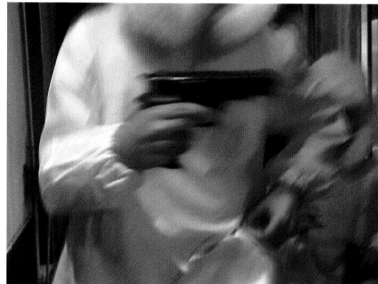
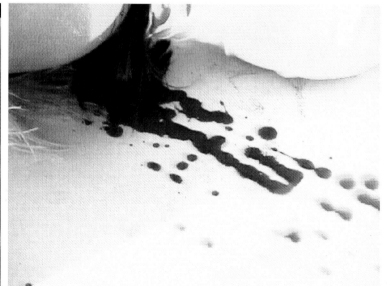
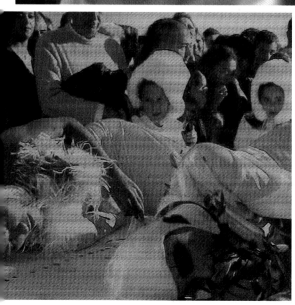
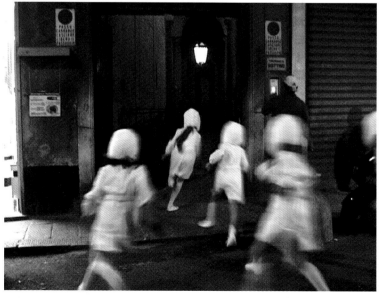

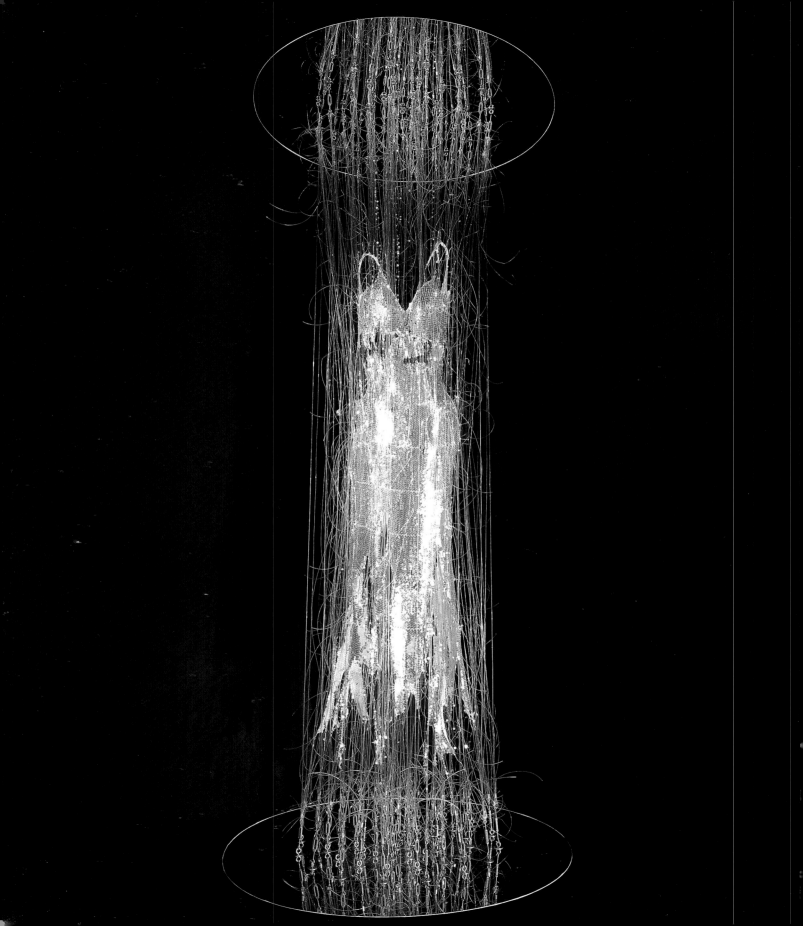

spectacle of yourself. Indeed, to be a self you may have to be a spectacle, and that is precisely what the little girls, slipping away from the massacre, continue to resist.

Kaoru and Starr offer particularly corporeal analogues of fashion's death; stark realizations of both a violent desire and desire for violence which inhabits fashion. By contrast, E. V. Day's *Transporter*, 1999, despite its material dissolution of the object, seems to promise a certain quietude, an entry into a peaceful, placatory sublime, rather than the terrifying intrusion of reality into our oneiric distancing from the world. *Transporter* is a Stephen Sprouse evening dress, its silvery, metallic fabric razored into thin strips, then, still loosely conforming to the shape of a body, suspended in a shaft of light. The 'transporter' of the title is a lift from *Star Trek*, the idea of the body being taken apart in one place and identically reassembled in another. Day's dress is a promise of evanescence, poised between here and elsewhere, between presence and absence. The gown looks, to appropriate the term to the vernacular, 'sublime': in its destruction, as remains in light, the dress is perhaps more nearly 'sublime' than when fully constituted. And almost whole, *Transporter* is a hole through which we are invited to enter the sublime, to return the term to philosophy and aesthetics. We are poised on the edge of a narrative of fragmentation, contemplating something which looks like that ultimate failure of language outlined by Lacan: this is an (in)essential object which isn't an object any longer. The dress occupies a perfect borderline position in which it is always *just* there, between reality and nothingness, between objectivity and intangible

recollection. This evanescence is perhaps how we would like to live: already 'dead' but perpetually suspended and protected from death. As Blanchot puts it, 'All that remains is the feeling of lightness that is death itself or, to put it more precisely, the instant of my death henceforth always in abeyance.'[8]

The tranquillity that *Transporter* evokes, however, is achieved at the cost of a carefully measured violence against the object of fashion, and, by implication, against a body for which it is surrogate. *Transporter* is a tantalizing embodiment of fashion's promise to defeat death, through perpetual change, through personal transformation. An embodiment, too, of its paradox: that in our resistance to death we wear what Hirosi calls 'this Death upon our backs'.[9] *Scarlet Aorta*, 2002, makes explicit this violence, the prophylactic death that guards against the intrusion of reality. Three scarlet evening gowns, with accompanying gloves, chokers and underwear, are assaulted and shredded. Where the quietude of *Transporter* arises in part from the concealment of its structure, here the monofilaments are no longer transparent, but rather a deep red, like jets of blood that radiate out of the forms, creating a tension which tears at the fabric. The intertwined forms are possessed of what Day calls a 'violent sanguinary energy', as if they were being torn apart by force – perhaps machine-gunned, or, as Day suggests, torn by a more remote, less certain power. 'The body in the dress is being ripped out with supernatural force, as unnatural and traumatic as it would be to rip the human psyche out of its relation to fashion.'[10] Pressed, Day comes up with a cinematic analogy and a striking aesthetic claim. The artist compares the narrative that

she reads into her work to the final scene of Vincent Gallo's *Buffalo 66* (1998), in which the male lead's death is shown in a slow-motion rotation (the dynamic which informs the three figures of *Scarlet Aorta*), with blood pulsing out of his skull. Day describes the scene as 'beautiful'. And in a sense, despite its horror, she is right: it is just that beauty is not a strong enough word for the blend of awful fascination and shock that the event creates. This is a point where the word, where language, including that of fashion to which art has so often and usefully had recourse, fails – or, as Day would have it, is torn apart by the tensions of antagonistic structures. What renders *Scarlet Aorta* is perhaps metaphorical for the larger relationship of art and fashion at the beginning of a new century.

Day's installations are 'dead' specimens – fashion rendered unwearable – which stand in the space of absent bodies. And yet, in the borderline between coherence and disintegration they live on, projecting themselves as ruin, endlessly into the future. *Transporter* and *Scarlet Aorta* are in the tradition of art's reaches into experience too beautiful, too terrifying, too violent to be commanded by coherent language. Turner was here; Rothko, too, but also, more disturbingly, Masson and Bellmer. Day's strategy is to reiterate those ventures into and back from the spiritual and sexual unknown with debased and denigrated materials of contemporary 'beauty'. Her violence edges the domestication of the picturesque back towards the inexpressible that fashion and art yearn for. Through the fragmentation of coherent signification, Day shifts both into an experiential and terminal domain ●

E. V. Day
Transporter, 2000
Silver sequin dress with monofilament, turnbuckles and mirrored disks

Always on the verge of being there, always on the threshold of disappearance, the (in)essential object of fashion is no longer an object, but rather symbolizes the evanescence of fashion and its promises, and ultimately of the body which it addresses.

Art and fashion: what common traits? That each begins in the register of the personal and terminates in the social. That this displacement is effected by an entropic debilitation of the individual vision. That each somehow believes in a utopia (or dystopia), whether in the image of the body perfected through design, or through the impossible prolepsis of art – the world as it should be wedged between the signifiers of the world as it is. This commonality fostered a relationship of sorts. For art, fashion was, for a while, a very useful way of talking about the world. Indeed, it constituted an escape route from art's self-negation. That negatory moment perhaps took a long time coming: we might even understand it as a condition of modernism which is only realized in the register of postmodernity.

From the mid-nineteenth century onwards, art, under pressure both from the transformations of its economic systems and from the novel embodiment of perspectival representation in the mechanical and chemical developments of the age – first the camera and then cinema – came to be as much about the scrutiny of its own use of a specific language as what was represented with that language. The French philosopher Jean-François Lyotard suggested that photography – because of its mechanical replication of the concept of perspectival vision – accepts the rules of the formation of pictural images as given and simply applies them. Lyotard understood the task of painting, robbed of its representational function in the wake of photography, to be the search for those rules of the formation of the image.[1] Just as mechanical reproduction has a complex engagement with painting that precedes the invention of chemical-mechanical photography in the 1830s, so perhaps we might understand that this undermining of

painting's language is not wholly a phenomenon of modernity, that it might indeed be a consequence, in itself, of perspectival conventions. However, as T. J. Clark points out, there is a crisis of representation which is manifest in the modern era. 'Something decisive happened in the history of art around Manet which set painting and the other arts on a new course. Perhaps the change can be described as a kind of scepticism, or at least unsureness, as to the nature of representation in art. There had been degrees of doubt on this subject before, but they had mostly appeared as asides to the central task of constructing a likeness, and in a sense they had guaranteed that task, making it seem all the more necessary and grand.'[2]

By the late 1960s and the early '70s, this scepticism towards its own language had so suffused art's practices that not only was representation negated, but the debate that modernism initiated had foreclosed itself through the intractability of its own language. The forms no longer seemed to exist through which to investigate the rules of representation: post-minimalist art in particular seemed to dwell on the impossibility of its own being. Whilst the art object no longer had the capacity to communicate this dilemma to a wider audience, far less provide a dialectical resolution, it continued to embody directly the old modernist discourse between socially transformative value and the formal insistence on *l'art pour l'art*. For accompanying this ideological nihilism was a paradoxical insistence on the apodicity of the art object's meaning, in a role whereby the artwork undertook a moral project first outlined for it by Diderot's insistence in the late eighteenth century upon an 'educational' and 'improving' content for art. Art's utopian vision was

no longer an impossible individual dream but imagined as something that was both collective and conceivable. Victor Burgin's analyses of the artefacts of popular culture, through the addition of 'instructive' texts, are paradigms of this pious virtue. The pedagogical imperative displaced what had been central tenets of art, even after the initiation of modernism's self-critique – narrative, formal questions of shape, colour and texture, and with those factors, the thorny issues of 'beauty' and visual pleasure. As Jeremy Gilbert-Rolfe observes, 'Much contemporary discourse is lodged in, or is the product of, a fear of pleasure. Which is to say, of instability, complexity, arousal without clear moral purpose.'[3]

Beauty and pleasure: words and concepts largely abandoned by art theory in the 1970s remain the stuff of fashion. Even when it is perverse, wilfully different and flagrantly in contravention of accepted tastes, fashion that works never does anything less than knock your eye out, never does anything more than arouse both wearer and spectator 'without clear moral purpose'. The rest is something for timid office types to wear for anonymity. Strangely enough, art used to work in this way, too. Visually the spectator was seduced, excited, enthralled, sometimes even – though it wasn't necessary – told a complex and important story (a story which, furthermore, didn't have to be true, any more than fashion tells the truth about its wearer). Dave Hickey, in a brief polemical treatise on beauty, maps out the consequences of art's retreat from seductive discourse into pedagogy. 'It was, after all, the invention of illusionistic space that bestowed upon the visual language of European culture those dimensions of "negativity" and "remote tense" that are generally taken to distinguish human languages from the languages of animals –

CONCLUSION

since these properties made it possible for us to lie and to imagine convincingly in our speech, to assert what we are denying and to construct narrative memory by contextualizing our assertions with regard to a past and a future, to a conditional or subjunctive reality. For four centuries visual culture in the West possessed these options – and exploited them. Today ... we remain content to slither through this flatland of Baudelairian modernity, trapped ... in the eternal, positive presentness of a terrain so visually impoverished that we cannot even lie to any effect in its language of images – nor imagine with any authority – nor even remember. And such is the Protestant hegemony of this anti-rhetorical flatness that contemporary artists have been, in effect, forced to divert their endeavours into realms of speech, dance, text, photography and installation design in order to exploit the semantic spaces and rhetorical felicities that are still available in literary and theatrical practice – so they might, at last, crudely approximate effects that were effortlessly available to Titian on his worst day.'[4]

One of the forms that artists sought as a recourse to art's nullification of its own language was fashion. Not fashion as fashion, but rather fashion as object of popular culture; fashion as source of formal languages with which to readdress the subjects of art – shape, colour and texture, 'beauty' and visual pleasure – from outside a closed linguistic field; and fashion as narrative – as a form which solicited its subjects, which seduced them through its formal and relational properties, and, as in the work of Sylvie Fleury and Elisa Jimenez, allowed a continual deferral of ending. Art and fashion were once both inherently seductive: fashion worn to seduce in an economy of erotic exchange, and, in

advance of that, seducing the economy of fiscal exchange. As Hickey divines, art could be equally inviting, equally capable of offering you a good time and not respecting you the following morning. Art and fashion: what common traits? Perhaps that both are (or were) good liars, because of the vitality of the utopias they promised, capable of signifying them in the complete absence of any concrete condition of any reality. What was more, as Hickey has also pointed out, elsewhere, in a 'marginal' text on popular culture,[5] audiences knew enough, recognizing contextual irony when they saw it, not to mind this duplicity, indeed accepting that their play within the process, their submission within the limited confines of the artwork, was a necessary part of the engagement with the image. Other than a cultural studies academic or a zealot, no one much expected art to utter a unified truth – but art's ever more engrossing solipsism meant that no one much, apart from zealous cultural studies academics, was any longer engaged with the image, and even then only as a text.

In a time of attenuation and proscription, fashion offered visual resources. An artist like Judith Shea, sensing the imminent collapse of art under the weight of its own introspection, could turn to it as a way of reviving those very properties that post-minimalism sought to eradicate. Shea was, of course, far from alone: the generation of artists that had grown up inside popular culture – the first TV generation – revelled in, more than reviled, the diversity of its imagery and meanings, even as, for example in the work of Cindy Sherman and Silvia Kolbowski, they rigorously tested its ideological implications. With this renewed vigour came satisfaction in looking. Kolbowski's 'Model Pleasure' series might have been

a thoroughly postmodern appreciation of woman's constitution in language, and Karen Kimmel's [open] is an incisive and witty scrutiny of the constitution and confirmation of social subjects, but neither observes any self-denying ordinances about refusing the pleasures of the spectator in the process. David Robbins, one of the leading American artists of the East Village avant-garde in the early 1980s has suggested that 'perhaps our most lasting contribution, intangible, but appearing everywhere since, may turn out to have been our restoration of a discourse of happiness, affirmation of the present and receptivity to the future, as an option for thinking artists'.[6] Indeed, one can trace the resonances of that avant-garde's embrace of popular culture – including the world of fashion – through the ambivalent affirmation of artists such as Kimmel, Alex Bag or Sylvie Fleury, to the sometimes less than critically balanced endorsements that emanated from Shoreditch and Hoxton in the 1990s.

However, there is a dissatisfaction. In the wake of art's own seduction by fashion, there is a sense that, whilst a temporary pleasure, those resources might not offer enough enduring and mutual interests to sustain the relationship. Robbins speaks of restoring art's 'receptivity to the future', and it is perhaps in the different time of objects within art and fashion, their duration and the mode of their cyclical return, that this difference becomes apparent. Silvia Kolbowski and Peter Eisenman's *Like the Difference between Autumn/Winter '94/'95 and Spring/Summer '95* is perhaps the most carefully considered appraisal of the incommensurability of temporalities, but elsewhere the tension surfaces in both a violence against beauty, as in the work of Graham Dolphin, and a beautiful violence, as in E. V. Day's carefully composed decompositions.

Have we escaped the moment of art's self-negation? The history of art in the last two decades suggests that at the least its grudging diminution of visual rhetoric and infelicitous pleasure is contested. That artists can turn and critique fashion, as Dolphin, Day, Izima Kaoru and Kirsten Glass do, might be a sign in itself of a diminished need for fashion as resource and refuge, and might reflect a new faith in their rhetorical capacities, rather than a renewal of the challenge to the ideological and historical condition of the object. What we may have here is not one of those repetitions and extensions of modernism's practice effected within postmodernism, to which Hal Foster points[7] – albeit one that would here be wholly framed by postmodernity – but rather a larger-scale cyclicality, a return to art as a seductive narrational language, telling its spectators a story about history and culture. If this return to language is a characteristic of art now, and is likely to characterize its future practice, then we may see an abandonment of those rhetorical devices, including fashion, to which artists have resorted. To an extent fashion will have done its job, as shelter, but ultimately it may represent a language that is not complex enough to compose the work of art as analysis and expression of the individual in history.

A difficulty of, rather than with, language may have its own set of implications, consequential for those who would spectate upon or regulate culture, rather than participate in it. The acceptance of a pious, morally weighted value for art has been accompanied by a massive expansion in its display, and in its exegeses. If art now returns to a discourse of difficulty – of being tough to explain or understand – partly because what is being said doesn't

have to be presented as or understood to be true; if it returns to a wilful, clever and cruel falsity in the context of its presentation while perhaps retaining and sharing fashion's seductive values, then there are several immediate possibilities. Perhaps there develops a creative and critical community that is grounded in history and cultural objects. What we have had for the last thirty years is one that promulgates a connection of objects to history through an a priori model of how history works and how culture articulates its teleology. It starts with theory and, jackdaw-like, appropriates and selectively reads those objects it chooses as most suitable to explain its beliefs. An alternative community has always (just about) existed, even as the business of art's interpretation has become bureaucratized and academicized. You will find its practitioners in artists' studios rather than scholastic conferences, engaged in the difficult business of looking at and writing about art rather than reading theory, making work rather than filling in grant application forms.

One alternative is that the difficulty of art becomes its own spectacle. As Hickey has recently written, art's visual attributes become the means by which we distinguish it from the spectacle of mass-mediated forms such as narrative cinema. 'We know it's art because we don't understand it and don't plan to try.'[8] Another possibility is that the objects of mass-media culture become the subject of an inflated discourse because they can be explained in – or rather more often endowed with – the terms which were once the domain of art criticism. This is, perhaps, the route by which fashion would maintain its recent relationship to art – shifting from a shared language of

practice to an appropriated language of explanation. It is this that would sustain the relationship of the last two decades, but on different terms. Such a strategy has allowed much fashion photography of the last five years to be the subject of critical programmes which have interpreted it not as an object of popular culture with something relevant to say about that culture, but as objects of art, made according to a vision in which the image's purpose in selling something was at best secondary and often wholly incidental. An example here would be the gallery exhibition of Steven Meisel's portfolio featuring Amber Valletta and Georgina Grenville for Versace's 2001 collections, described in the accompanying press release as recalling 'the Mannerist portraits of Bronzino and Pontormo where the sumptuously adorned female subjects are both hieratic and untouchable'.[9] Which may be true, but I don't think that either Bronzino or Pontormo had a primary goal of selling exclusive, beautiful garments, even if, like Meisel, they were trying to keep a powerful patron happy. A parallel, if reversed, strategy is to interpret that which is difficult – art meditated, both formally and thematically challenging – in terms only of the sensation that accompanies its reception and sometimes – artists and curators being no fools when it comes to claiming attention – its presentation. Typical of this is the popular discourse that surrounds artists as diverse, and difficult, as Tracey Emin and Jeff Koons. For fashion, what is made as an object of pleasure is promoted as profound (perhaps because we still lack the tools to apprehend those of its components that pleasure us). For art (perhaps through a similar lack), what is made as an object of profundity is understood as simply pleasurable, and trivial, spectacle.

INTRODUCTION

1. Gilbert-Rolfe, J., 'A Thigh-Length History of the Fashion Photograph – An Abbreviated History of the Body' in *Beyond Piety: Critical Essays on the Visual Arts* (Cambridge: Cambridge University Press: 1995), p. 261
2. Freud, S., (1940 [1922]), 'The Medusa's Head' in *The Standard Edition of the Complete Psychological Works of Sigmund Freud Vol. XVIII*, (London: Hogarth Press: 1955), p. 273
3. Hickey, D., *Enter the Dragon: Four Essays on Beauty* (San Francisco: Art Issues Press: 1993), p. 16
4. Benjamin, W., *The Arcades Project*, Convolutes B [Fashion] (Cambridge, MA: The Bellknap Press of Harvard University Press: 1999), p. 62
5. Barth, J., *Chimera* (London: André Deutsch: 1974)
6. Lacan, J., *The Seminar of Jacques Lacan: Book II, The Ego in Freud's Theory and in the Technique of Psychoanalysis, 1954–55* (New York: W. W. Norton: 1988), p. 164
7. ibid.

1 CONCEPTUALISM AND FASHION'S REJECTION

1. Alberro, A., 'The Dialectics of Everyday Life: Martha Rosler and the Strategy of the Decoy' in de Zegher, C. (ed.), *Martha Rosler: Positions in the Life World* (Cambridge, MA: M.I.T Press: 1998), p. 76
2. Fox, H. N., 'Waiting in the Wings: Desire and Destiny in the Art of Eleanor Antin' in Fox, H. N. (ed.), *Eleanor Antin* (Los Angeles: Los Angeles County Museum of Art: 1999), p. 44
3. Behr, E., 'Introduction' in Newton, H., *Sleepless Nights* (London: Quartet Books: 1978), p. 6
4. Brooks, R., 'Brutality Chic', *ZG* No. 2, 1980, np.
5. ibid.
6. Conversation with the artist, August 2001
7. Brooks, R., 'Duggie Fields: Interview', *ZG* No. 1, 1980, np.

2 AMBIVALENT EMBRACE

1. Conversation with the author, December 2000
2. Cartledge, F., 'Dress to Impress? Local punk fashion and commodity exchange' in Sabin, R. (ed.), *Punk Rock: So What? The Cultural Legacy of Punk* (London: Routledge: 1999), pp. 144-5
3. Conversation with the author, December 2000

4. *The Face*, October 1984, p. 34
5. *Harpers & Queen*, January 2001, p. 66
6. Liebmann, L., 'Cindy Sherman: Metro Pictures', *Artforum* XXII, No. 7 (March 1984), p. 95
7. ibid.
8. Schjeldhal, P., *Cindy Sherman*, (New York: Whitney Museum of American Art: 1987), p. 11
9. Owens, C., 'Posing' in *Beyond Recognition: Representation, Power, and Culture* (Berkeley: University of California Press: 1992), pp. 213-14

3 THE EMPTY BODY PART 1

1. Coplans, J., 'My Chronology' in *A Self-Portrait* (New York: PS1/DAP: 1998), p. 134. The artist in question was Lucas Samaras.
2. Sischy, I. and Celant, G., 'Editorial', *Artforum* XX, No. 6 (February 1982), p. 34
3. ibid.
4. ibid., p. 35
5. Blau, H., *Nothing in Itself: Complexions of Fashion* (Bloomington: Indiana University Press: 1999), p. 22
6. Bénaim, L., *Issey Miyake* (London: Thames & Hudson: 1997), p. 17
7. Krane, S., *Lynda Benglis: Dual Natures* (Atlanta: High Museum of Art: 1991), p. 24
8. Sischy and Celant, op cit, p. 35
9. Barthes, R., *Camera Lucida* (London: Vintage Books: 1993), p. 51
10. Derrida, J., 'Foreword: *Fors*: The Anglish Words of Nicolas Abraham and Maria Torok' in Abraham, N. and Torok, M., *The Wolf Man's Magic Word: A Cryptonymy* (Minneapolis: University of Minnesota Press: 1986)
11. Letter to the author, August 2001
12. ibid.
13. Krane, op cit.
14. Steele, V., 'The Corset: Fashion and Eroticism', *Fashion Theory* Vol. 3, No. 2 (December 1999), p. 473

4 THE EMPTY BODY PART 2

1. Foote, N., 'The Apotheosis of the Crummy Space', *Artforum* XV, No. 2 (October 1976)
2. Flood, R., 'Essay on Judith Shea' in *Seven Artists* (New York: State University of New York/Neuberger Museum: 1980), p. 39
3. Raynor, V., 'Art: Two Women Take Crafts to Higher Plane', *New York Times*, 27 June 1980

4. Silverthorne, J., 'Judith Shea', *Artforum* XIX, No. 2 (October 1980)
5. Cohen, R. H., 'Judith Shea at Willard', *Art in America* (October 1980), p. 130
6. Quoted in *Figuratively Speaking: Drawings by Seven Artists* (New York: Neuberger Museum: 1989), p. 88
7. Krauss, R., 'Sculpture in the Expanded Field' in *The Originality of the Avant-Garde and Other Modernist Myths* (Cambridge, MA: M.I.T Press: 1985), p. 279
8. Schjeldhal, P., 'Judith Shea: Monument Statuary', *Village Voice*, 16 April 1991, p. 99

5 FRAGMENTS OF FASHION

1. Gilbert-Rolfe, op cit, p. 259
2. Derrida, op cit, p. xiv
3. Metz, C., 'Photography and Fetish', *October* 34 (Fall 1985), p. 85
4. Derrida, op cit, p. xvii
5. Fuss, D., *Identification Papers* (London: Routledge: 1995), p. 1
6. Freud, S., 'Group Psychology and the Analysis of the Ego' in *Penguin Freud Library Vol. 12 (Civilisation, Society and Religion)* (London: Penguin Books: 1985), pp. 134-40
7. Freud, S. (1917), 'Mourning and Melancholia' in *The Standard Edition of the Complete Psychological Works of Sigmund Freud Vol. XIV*, (London: Hogarth Press: 1957), p. 249
8. Lacan, J., *Le Séminaire de Jacques Lacan: Livre XI, Les quatre concepts fondamentaux de la psychanalyse* (Paris: Editions de Seuil: 1973), p. 219 (author's translation)
9. Fogle, D. and Wilcox, T. J., 'Interview' in *T. J. Wilcox* (London: ICA/Gavin Brown's Enterprise: 1998), np.
10. ibid.

6 SHOPPING IN SPACE

1. The editors of *October*, 'Introduction', *October: The First Decade, 1976-1986* (Cambridge, MA: M.I.T Press: 1987), p. x
2. See Deutsche, R. and Ryan, C. G., 'The Fine Art of Gentrification', *October* 31 (Fall 1984), pp. 91-111
3. Martin, R., *Architectures of Display* (New York: 1995). Project leaflet, np.
4. ibid.

5. O'Brien, G., 'Like Art', *Artforum* XXIV, No. 9 (May 1988), p. 18
6. Interview with Nick Cross, Marketing Director of Selfridges, August 2000
7. O'Brien, G., 'Into the Gap: Art Club 2000', *Artforum* XXXII, No. 6 (February 1994), p. 75
8. Kolbowski, S., *Closed Circuit* (New York: Postmasters Gallery: 1997), p. 5

7 FORM AND UNIFORM

1. Muelhig, L., 'Big Silver' in *Beverly Semmes* (West Palm Beach: Norton Museum of Art: 1996), p. 7
2. ibid
3. Crutchfield, M., 'The Presence of Absence' in *Beverly Semmes* (West Palm Beach: Norton Museum of Art: 1996), p. 17
4. Veshard, J., 'Buy-O-Sphere', *Madison*, January/February 2000, p. 78
5. Horodner, S., 'Helpful Measures', *Surface* 13, 1998, np.
6. ibid.

8 DRESSING UP DRESSING DOWN

1. Letter to the author, October 2001
2. ibid
3. See Currie, E., 'Prescribing Fashion: Dress, Politics and Gender in Early 16th Century Conduct Literature' in *Fashion Theory*, Vol. 4, No. 2 (June 2000), pp. 157-78, and Bell, R. M., *How to Do It: Guides to Good Living for Renaissance Italians* (Chicago: Chicago University Press: 1999)
4. Weber, M. and The Creative Design Group, *Dress Casually for Success for Men* (New York: McGraw Hill: 1997)
5. Conversation with the artist, April 2001
6. Letter from the artist, October 2001
7. Conversation with the artist, April 2001
8. 'Mediastine' is an obsolete noun used in the sixteenth to eighteenth centuries to describe menial kitchen workers and domestic drudges. An era of low-paid, or unpaid, entry-level jobs for those aspiring to media careers is perhaps the appropriate historical moment to revive the term with a new specificity of role and equivalence of status.

9 WHO WILL YOU BE TODAY?

1. Hughes, A., *Nylon* 058 (May 2000), np.

2. Quoted in *Dutch* 27, June 2000, np.
3. Chaplin, J., 'You're a "Beamer," She Said, And Picked Me To Model', *New York Times*, 3 October 1999, Section 9, p. 8
4. Lippard, L., *Overlay: Contemporary Art and the Art of Prehistory* (New York: Pantheon: 1983), p. 46
5. Jimenez often barters dresses for other services within the artistic and fashion communities. Conversation with the author, May 2001.
6. Cited in Hughes, op cit.

10 NOT CUT TO PATTERN

1. For such an appraisal see Stallabrass, J., *High Art Lite* (London: Verso: 1999)
2. Clark, T. J., *The Painting of Modern Life: Paris in the Art of Manet and his Followers* (London: Thames & Hudson: 1984), p. 253
3. Stallabrass, op cit. p. 134

11 TO DIE FOR

1. Kracauer, S., 'Photography' in *The Mass Ornament: Weimar Essays* (Cambridge, MA: Harvard University Press: 1995), pp. 50-51
2. Blanchot, M. (1989), 'The Work and Death's Space' in *The Space of Literature* (Lincoln: University of Nebraska Press: 1989), p. 122
3. ibid., p. 103
4. Jones, A., 'Dario Argento', *Cinefantastique*, Vol. 18, No. 2/3 (March 1988)
5. Hirosi, O., 'Izima Kaoru's Aesthetic of the Baroque Figure' in *Kaoru sitai no aru 20 no hûkei* (Tokyo: Korinsha Press: 1999), np.
6. ibid.
7. Hagenberg, R., 'Facing Death: Izima Kaoru's "20 Landscapes with a Corpse"' in *Kaoru sitai no aru 20 no hûkei*, op cit.
8. Blanchot, M. (2000), *The Instant of My Death* (San Francisco: Stanford University Press: 2000), p. 11
9. Hirosi, op cit.
10. Conversation with the author, December 2001

CONCLUSION

1. Lyotard, J.-F., *The Inhuman: Reflections on Time* (Cambridge: Polity Press: 1991), pp. 120-21
2. Clark, op cit., p. 10

3. Gilbert-Rolfe, J., 'Nonrepresentation in 1988: Meaning-Production Beyond the Scope of the Pious' in *Beyond Piety: Critical Essays on the Visual Arts* (Cambridge: Cambridge University Press: 1995), p. 53
4. Hickey, D., *The Invisible Dragon: Four Essays on Beauty* (Los Angeles: Art Issues Press: 1994), p. 40
5. Hickey, D., 'Pontormo's Rainbow' in *Air Guitar: Essays on Art and Democracy* (Los Angeles: Art Issues Press: 1997)
6. Robbins, D., 'ABC TV', *Artforum* XXXVIII, No. 2 (October 1999), p. 160
7. Foster, H., *The Return of the Real* (Cambridge, MA: M.I.T Press: 1996), pp. 71-96
8. Hickey, D., 'Little Victories' in *Frieze*, 63 (November/December 2001), p. 99
9. Press release for Steven Meisel exhibition, White Cube Gallery, London, 2001

PICTURE CREDITS

L = Left, C = Centre, R = Right, T = Top, B = Bottom
Measurements are given in centimetres followed by inches, height before width

pp. 6-7 Frank Moore, *To Die For*, 70.5 x 156.5 (27³/₄ x 61⁵/₈). Photo Tom Powel, courtesy the artist and Sperone Westwater, New York

p. 9L Andy Warhol dress (Marilyn), courtesy Versace

p. 9R Gold Medusa watch, courtesy Versace

p. 11 Chris Ofili, *Absolut Ofili*. Permission of V & S Vin & Sprit AB/Absolut Vodka

p. 12 inset Silvia Kolbowski and Peter Eisenman, *Like the Difference between Autumn/Winter '94/'95 and Spring/Summer '95*. Photo Michael Moran and Silvia Kolbowski, courtesy Silvia Kolbowski and Kenneth Frampton

p. 12 Helmut Lang store. Photo Paul Warchol, courtesy Gluckman Mayner Architects

p. 13 Helmut Lang Parfumerie. Photo Lydia Gould, courtesy Gluckman Mayner Architects

p. 14 Mary Boone Gallery, New York. Courtesy Gluckman Mayner Architects

p. 15 Gagosian Gallery, New York. Courtesy Gluckman Mayner Architects

p. 17 Judith Shea, *King* 152.4 x 63.5 (60 x 25); *Queen* 182.9 x 182.9 (72 x 72). Courtesy Herbert and Dorothy Vogel Collection, New York

p. 19 Suit, courtesy Ann Demeulemeester and Michele Montagne

p. 20 White keyhole dress, courtesy Gucci

p. 25 Victor Burgin, *Lei-feng*, 40.6 x 50.8 (16 x 20). Photo © Tate, London 2002

p. 26 Victor Burgin, *St Laurent demands a whole new life style*, 89 x 129 (35 x 50³/₄). Courtesy L. and M. Galerie Durand-Dessert, Paris

p. 28L Martha Rosler, *Untitled (S, M, L)*, 50.8 x 40.5 (20 x 16). Courtesy Anne de Villepoix and the artist

p. 28R Martha Rosler, *Untitled (Isn't it nice to feel feminine again)*. Courtesy Anne de Villepoix and the artist

p. 29 Eleanor Antin, *Representational Painting*. Courtesy Electronic Arts Intermix, New York

p. 30 Hannah Wilke, *Super-T-Art*, 101.6 x 81.3 (40 x 32). Photo D. James Dee, courtesy Ronald Feldman Fine Arts, © Scharlatt Family

p. 31 Helmut Newton, *Office Love*. © Helmut Newton/Maconochie Photography

p. 32L Helmut Newton, *From the Story of Ohhh*. © Helmut Newton/Maconochie Photography

p. 32R Helmut Newton, *Store Dummies 1*. © Helmut Newton/Maconochie Photography

p. 33 Helmut Newton, *Maxim's 1*. © Helmut Newton/Maconochie Photography

pp. 34-5 General Idea, *File* cover and spread. Photos Jo Broughton, courtesy Duggie Fields, © A. A. Bronson

p. 36 Duggie Fields, *Modes of Perception*, 182.9 x 182.9 (72 x 72). Photo Prudence Cuming Associates, courtesy the artist

p. 37 Duggie Fields, *Just a Chance Encounter and Goodness Knows What Complications May Follow*, 223.5 x 203.2 (88 x 80). Photo Prudence Cuming Associates, courtesy the artist

p. 42 Dianne Blell, *Two Women Discovering Urban Cupid*, each framed print 20.3 x 25.4 (8 x 10). Photo Michael Tighe, courtesy the artist

p. 43 Dianne Blell, *Young Woman Overtaken by a Storm*, each print 43.2 x 35.6 (17 x 14). Photo EDO, courtesy the artist

p. 44 Shari Dienes, T-shirt. Photo Tom Warren, courtesy Stefan Eins, © Fashion Moda

p. 44C Kano, jacket. Photo Humberto Lopez, courtesy Kate Shanley

p. 44B Jenny Holzer, baseball cap. Photo Jo Broughton, courtesy Bob Bentley

p. 45 Jenny Holzer, T-shirt. Photo Tom Warren, courtesy Stefan Eins, © Fashion Moda

p. 46L Keith Haring, T-shirts. Photo Lisa Kahane, courtesy Stefan Eins, © Fashion Moda

p. 46C Katherine Hamnett, T-shirt. Courtesy P A Photos

p. 46R Tracey Emin and Sarah Lucas, T-shirt. Courtesy Sadie Coles HQ, © Sarah Lucas

pp. 46-7 Stefan Eins, T-shirt. Photo Tom Warren, courtesy Stefan Eins, © Fashion Moda

pp. 48-9 'Urban Scrawl', courtesy *Harpers & Queen*/National Magazine Company, © Masoud

p. 51 Jean Michel Basquiat, *A Panel of Experts*, 152.4 x 152.4 (60 x 60). © ADAGP, Paris & DACS, London 2002

p. 53L Cindy Sherman, *Untitled # 119*. Courtesy the artist and Metro Pictures

p. 53R Cindy Sherman, *Untitled # 132*. Courtesy the artist and Metro Pictures

p. 55 Silvia Kolbowksi, *Model Pleasure VIII*, each photo 20.3 x 25.4 (8 x 10). Courtesy American Fine Arts and the artist

p. 59 *Artforum* cover. Photo Jo Broughton (cover photo Eiichiro Sakata), courtesy *Artforum*

p. 60 Abura-gami coat. Photo Tsutomu Wakatuki, courtesy Issey Miyake

p. 61 Lynda Benglis, *Untitled*. Courtesy the artist/ © VAGA, New York & DACS, London 2002

p. 63L Maureen Connor, *Inside Out*, 99 x 71.1 x 88.9 (39 x 28 x 35). Photo Steven Sloman, courtesy the artist

p. 63C Maureen Connor, *Undertitled*, 88.9 x 61 x 38.1 (35 x 24 x 15). Photo Steven Sloman, courtesy the artist

p. 63R Wire body. Photo Daniel Jouanneau, courtesy Issey Miyake

p. 64 Zizi Raymond, *Untitled (Undertow)*, 73.7 x 45.7 x 5.1 (29 x 18 x 2). Courtesy Craig and Laada Ruse

p. 65L Zizi Raymond, *Hiding*, 167.6 x 233.7 x 40.6 (66 x 92 x 16). Courtesy the artist

p. 65R Maureen Connor, *Birth of the Bustle*, 111.8 x 83.8 x 40.6 (44 x 33 x 16). Photo Steven Sloman, courtesy the artist

p. 66L Classique fragrances. Courtesy Kenneth Green Associates, © Jean Paul Gaultier

p. 66R Madonna in Gaultier corset. Photo Fitzroy Barrett, courtesy Retna Pictures Ltd

p. 67 'Nymphs' dress. Photo Ugo Camera, courtesy Vivienne Westwood, © Ugo Camera

p. 69 Julie Major, *Untitled (after Gabrielle d'Estrées and her sister)*, 63 x 66 x 45 (24³/₄ x 26 x 17³/₄). Private collection

p. 73 Chloë Sevigny modelling Martin Margiela. Photos courtesy Mark Borthwick

p. 74 Judith Shea, 'Black and White Jacket' series, studio view. Photo courtesy the artist

p. 75 Judith Shea, *New Urban Landscape # 9*. Photo Jonathan Dent, courtesy Institute for Art and Urban Resources, New York

p. 76T Judith Shea, "Judy", 63.5 x 61 (25 x 24); "Peggy", 43.2 x 53.3 (17 x 21); "Kathy", 54.6 x 55.9 (21¹/₂ x 22). Photo courtesy the artist

p. 76B Judith Shea, *Black Jacket*, 63.5 x 63.5 (25 x 25). Photo courtesy the artist

p. 77 Judith Shea, *Black Dress*, 113 x 38.1 x 30.5 (44¹/₂ x 15 x 12). Courtesy Raymond Learsy Collection, New York

p. 78 Judith Shea, *Shield*, 182.9 x 38.1 x 38.1 (72 x 15 x 15). Photo courtesy the artist

p. 79 Judith Shea, *Eden*, coat 156.2 x 81.3 x 38.1 (61¹/₂ x 32 x 15); dress 143.5 x 40.6 x 27.9 (56¹/₂ x 16 x 11). Photo courtesy the artist

p. 83 Karen Kilimnick, *High Cheekbones*, 88.9 x 58.4 (35 x 23). Courtesy the artist and emily Tsingou gallery

p. 84 Karen Kilimnick, *Curried and Immaculate*, 101.6 x 66 (40 x 26). Courtesy the artist and emily Tsingou gallery

pp. 86-7 T. J. Wilcox, photographs from the film *The Escape (of Marie Antoinette)*, 40.6 x 50.8 (16 x 20). Courtesy the artist and Metro Pictures

p. 88 T. J. Wilcox, *Stephen Tennant Hommage*, 50.8 x 40.6 (20 x 16). Courtesy the artist and Metro Pictures

pp. 92-3 Silvia Kolbowski and Peter Eisenman, *Like the Difference between Autumn/Winter '94/'95 and Spring/Summer '95*. Photos Michael Moran and Silvia Kolbowski, courtesy Silvia Kolbowski and Kenneth Frampton

p. 95 Suit; suit with full skirt; cap-sleeved asymmetric coat-dress; long dress, all courtesy Comme des Garçons

p. 97 Vanessa Beecroft, *Show*. Courtesy the artist and Deitch Projects

p. 98 Courtesy Patrick Gries for Fondation Cartier pour l'art contemporain, Paris

pp. 98-9 Sam Taylor-Wood, *XV Seconds*. Photo Merley von Sternberg, courtesy the artist and Selfridges

p. 101T Art Club 2000, *Untitled (Times Square/Gap Grunge 2)*, 50.8 x 61 (20 x 24). Courtesy American Fine Arts

p. 101B Art Club 2000, *Untitled (Conran's 1)*, 20.3 x 25.4 (8 x 10). Courtesy American Fine Arts

p. 104T Beverly Semmes, *Big Silver*, dimensions variable. Courtesy the artist and Leslie Tonkonow Artworks and Projects, New York. Collection Irish Museum of Modern Art, Dublin

p. 104B Beverly Semmes, *Red Dress*, 386 x 320 x 1386.8 (152 x 126 x 546). Photo Patricia Wallace, courtesy the artist and Leslie Tonkonow Artworks and Projects, New York. Collection Hirshhorn Museum and Sculpture Garden, Washington, D.C.

p. 105L Beverly Semmes, *Haze*, ca. 366 x 282 (ca. 144 x 111). Courtesy the artist and Leslie Tonkonow Artworks and Projects, New York. Collection Hirshhorn Museum and Sculpture Garden, Washington, D.C.

p. 105R Beverly Semmes, *Watching Her Feat*, created in collaboration with The Fabric Workshop and Museum, PA, dimensions variable. Photo Aaron Igler, courtesy the artist and Leslie Tonkonow Artworks and Projects, New York

p. 108T Karen Kimmel, *[open]*, two performers. Photo Yvonne Venega, courtesy the artist and Sara Meltzer Gallery

p. 108BL Karen Kimmel, *[open]*, Appraiser equipment. Photo Herman Feldhaus, courtesy the artist and Sara Meltzer Gallery

p. 108BR Karen Kimmel, *[open]*, one performer. Photo Yvonne Venega, courtesy the artist and Sara Meltzer Gallery

p. 109 Karen Kimmel, *[open]*, installation view. Photo Herman Feldhaus, courtesy the artist and Sara Meltzer Gallery

p. 114 Maureen Connor, *Copy Room*. Courtesy the artist

p. 115TL Maureen Connor, *Conference Room*. Courtesy the artist

p. 115CL Maureen Connor, *Flying Clothes 2*. Courtesy the artist

p. 115BL Maureen Connor, *Tired*. Courtesy the artist

p. 115TR Maureen Connor, sartorial codes table from *Dress Down Friday*. Courtesy the artist

p. 115BR From A. Hunt, *Governance of the Consuming Passions – A History of Sumptuary Laws* (Basingstoke: Macmillan: 1996). By kind permission of the publishers

pp. 116-17 Karin Schaefer, *Lunula*, 243.8 x 61 x 61 (96 x 24 x 24). Photos Myriam Babin, courtesy the artist

p. 119 Charles LeDray, *Untitled*, 51.4 x 32.4 x 10.2 (20¼ x 12¾ x 4). Photo Oren Slor, courtesy Sperone Westwater, New York. Collection Kimberly Light, Pasadena

p. 120T Alex Bag, *Untitled (The Fashion Show)*. Courtesy the artist and P.H.A.G. Inc.

p. 120B Alex Bag, *Untitled (White Radio Girls)*. Courtesy the artist and P.H.A.G. Inc.

p. 124 Sylvie Fleury, *Agent Provocateur*, dimensions variable. Courtesy Laure Genillard/the artist

p. 125 Sylvie Fleury, *Moisturizing is the Answer*, 14 x 250 (5½ x 98⅜). Photo Jens Ziehe, Berlin, courtesy Chouakri Brahms Berlin, Berlin

pp. 128-9 Elisa Jimenez, working drawings for performance, each 29.7 x 21 (11⅝ x 8¼). Courtesy the artist

p. 130 Elisa Jimenez, working drawing for mirror installation. Courtesy the artist

p. 131 *bag people*, courtesy Saskia Draxler, Johannes Buss and Mona Kuschel, © High End Performance Art Projekt

p. 134 Maureen Paley. Photo Edina van der Wyck, courtesy Edina van der Wyck and Maureen Paley. © *Vogue*, Condé Nast Publications Ltd, London

p. 135 Tracey Emin/Vivienne Westwood. Photos Mat Collishaw, courtesy Vivienne Westwood and Tracey Emin, © Vivienne Westwood

p. 136 Kate Moss *Vogue* cover. Photo Sarah Morris, courtesy the artist, © *Vogue*, Condé Nast Publications Ltd, London

p. 137 Sarah Morris, *KTMSS*, 256.5 x 198 (101 x 78). Photo Stephen White. Private collection, courtesy Ivor Braka Ltd, London

p. 138 Tracey Emin, Polaroid photos, 8.8 x 10.7 (3⁷⁄₁₆ x 4³⁄₁₆). Courtesy Jay Jopling/White Cube, London

p. 140 Marc Quinn, study for *Beauty*, 348 x 140 x 140 (137 x 55⅛ x 55⅛). Photo Robin Derrick, courtesy Jay Jopling/White Cube, London

p. 141 Marc Quinn, casting of *Beauty*. Photo Robin Derrick, courtesy Jay Jopling/White Cube, London

p. 143 Jake and Dinos Chapman, *Kate*, 30 x 18 (11⅞ x 7). Photo Robin Derrick, courtesy Jay Jopling/White Cube, London

p. 145 Duggie Fields, *Catwalk of Life*. Courtesy the artist and *Pop*

p. 146 Hannah Starkey, *Untitled – Vogue, August 1999*, 122 x 152 (48 x 60). Courtesy Maureen Paley, Interim Art, London

pp. 146-7 Hannah Starkey, *Untitled – March 1999*, 122 x 152 (48 x 60). Courtesy Saatchi Collection, London

p. 148T Henry Bond, *5012*, 100 x 140 (39⅜ x 55). Courtesy the artist and emily Tsingou gallery

p. 148B Henry Bond, *5021*, 100 x 140 (39⅜ x 55). Courtesy the artist and emily Tsingou gallery

p. 149 Henry Bond, *5022*, 100 x 140 (39⅜ x 55). Courtesy the artist and emily Tsingou gallery

p. 153TL Kirsten Glass, *Aerosoul*, 168 x 238 (66⅛ x 93⅝). Courtesy Laure Genillard

p. 153BL Kirsten Glass, *Ultra Low*, 168.2 x 237.8 (66⅛ x 93⅝). Courtesy Saatchi Collection, London

p. 153TR Kirsten Glass, *D. J. L.*, 50 x 60 (19⅝ x 23⅝). Photo Dennis Schoenberg, courtesy the artist

p. 153BR Kirsten Glass, *Christine*, 100 x 100 (39⅜ x 39⅜). Photo Dennis Schoenberg, courtesy Shez Dawood

p. 154TL Graham Dolphin, *Untitled (soldering iron drawing 27)*, 21 x 28 (8⅜ x 11). Courtesy the artist and *Elle* UK

p. 154CL Graham Dolphin, *Untitled (Frank, September 1998)*, 27 x 20 (10⅝ x 7⅞). Courtesy the artist and *Frank*

p. 154BL Graham Dolphin, *Untitled (Dazed & Confused, February 1999 – pinned)*, 22 x 29 (8⅝ x 11⅜). Courtesy the artist and *Dazed & Confused*

p. 154R Graham Dolphin, *Untitled (Frank, March 1999 – resin)*, 27 x 20 (10⅝ x 7⅞). Courtesy the artist and *Frank*

pp. 156-7 Izima Kaoru, *Kojima Hijiri wears Yohji Yamamoto 231–233*, 100 x 127 (39⅜ x 50). Courtesy the artist and fa projects, London

p. 159 Dario Argento's catwalk show for Trussardi Action. Courtesy Trussardi Archive

p. 161 Izima Kaoru, *Akikawa Risa wears Chanel 021*, 100 x 127 (39⅜ x 50). Courtesy the artist and fa projects, London

p. 162 Robert Longo, *# 41 Untitled*, 243.8 x 487.7 x 91.4 (96 x 192 x 36). Courtesy the artist and Metro Pictures

p. 163L Robert Longo, *D-12 Untitled*, 114.3 x 88.9 (45 x 35). Courtesy the artist and Metro Pictures

p. 163R Robert Longo, *D-53 Untitled*, 243.8 x 152.4 (96 x 60). Courtesy the artist and Metro Pictures

pp. 164-5 Georgina Starr, *The Bunny Lake Collection*, 173 x 213 (68⅛ x 83⅞). Courtesy the artist and emily Tsingou gallery

p. 166 E. V. Day, *Transporter*, 121.9 x 121.9 x 292.1 (48 x 48 x 115). Photo Ron Amstutz, courtesy Henry Urbach Architecture. Collection Anthony Podesta

With many thanks to all the artists, galleries, lenders and contributors

INDEX